The Busy Caregiver's Guide to
Advanced Alzheimer Disease

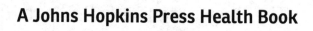
A Johns Hopkins Press Health Book

The Busy Caregiver's Guide to Advanced Alzheimer Disease

Jennifer R. Stelter, PsyD

With Rachael Wonderlin

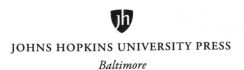

JOHNS HOPKINS UNIVERSITY PRESS

Baltimore

Note to the Reader: This book is not meant to substitute for medical care, and treatment should not be based solely on its contents. Instead, treatment must be developed in a dialogue between the individual and their physician. The book has been written to help with that dialogue.

© 2021 Johns Hopkins University Press
All rights reserved. Published 2021
Printed in the United States of America on acid-free paper
9 8 7 6 5 4 3 2 1

Johns Hopkins University Press
2715 North Charles Street
Baltimore, Maryland 21218-4363
www.press.jhu.edu

Library of Congress Cataloging-in-Publication Data

Names: Stelter, Jennifer R., 1978– author. | Wonderlin, Rachael, 1989– author.
Title: The busy caregiver's guide to advanced Alzheimer disease / Jennifer R.
    Stelter, PsyD, with Rachael Wonderlin.
Description: Baltimore : Johns Hopkins University Press, [2021] | Series: A Johns
    Hopkins Press health book | Includes bibliographical references and index.
Identifiers: LCCN 2020036318 | ISBN 9781421441078 (hardcover) |
    ISBN 9781421441085 (paperback) | ISBN 9781421441092 (ebook)
Subjects: LCSH: Alzheimer's disease—Patients—Care. | Caregivers. | Dementia—
    Patients—Care. | Alzheimer's disease—Patients—Family relationships.
Classification: LCC RC523 .S733 2021 | DDC 616.8/311—dc23
LC record available at https://lccn.loc.gov/2020036318

A catalog record for this book is available from the British Library.

The images on pages 5 and 10 are from Peter Rabins, *Is It Alzheimer's? 101 Answers to Your Most Pressing Questions about Memory Loss and Dementia* (Baltimore, MD: Johns Hopkins University Press, 2020). The images on pages 80 and 81 are from AdobeStock and iStockphoto.com, respectively. All other images are the author's.

Special discounts are available for bulk purchases of this book. For more information, please contact Special Sales at specialsales@jh.edu.

Johns Hopkins University Press uses environmentally friendly book materials, including recycled text paper that is composed of at least 30 percent post-consumer waste, whenever possible.

*To my children, Jack and Julianna, who helped me
see the vision for this model. Because of them,
writing this book was possible.*

Contents

Preface ix

Acknowledgments xiii

Chapter 1. What Is Alzheimer Disease? 1

Chapter 2. What Is the Dementia Connection Model? 17

Chapter 3. Using the Dementia Connection Model 29

Chapter 4. Communication Challenges 43

Chapter 5. Eating, Feeding, and Nutrition Challenges 55

Chapter 6. Sleeping Challenges 69

Chapter 7. Toileting Challenges 79

Chapter 8. Bathing Challenges 87

Chapter 9. Pain and Pain Management 97

Chapter 10. Depression, Hallucinations, and Delusions 105

Chapter 11. Repetitive Behavior, Rummaging, and Collecting 115

Chapter 12. Sundowning, Aggression, and Wandering 123

Chapter 13. Intentional Care 133

Chapter 14. Promoting Brain Health 141

References 151

Index 167

Preface

In this book, I introduce you to a three-pronged approach to dementia care, known as the Dementia Connection Model. This model, for the first time, ties together three known concepts in the dementia care field: retrogenesis, habilitation, and sensory-based knowledge. The goals of this book are to be completely transparent about what can happen as the disease progresses, assist you in better understanding what your loved one is experiencing, and explain how to connect to them in a meaningful way. I want you to feel the "win-win"!

My adventure in writing this book started after years of studying, creating, and using the Dementia Connection Model with my patients. I'm always in pursuit of the "why?" Why does this happen to us, why do the symptoms occur, why is there no cure, and so on. And not so much what happens as Alzheimer disease develops, because there is wonderful research out there supporting this information that should be reviewed. But more so of "Why does mom act this way?" or "Why can't dad do this anymore?" I know that in Western culture there is less pursuit of why things happen and more attention paid to treating symptoms, but I'm not good with that. I'm in pursuit of more. I truly feel that if a caregiver understands the "why?" they can then step into the shoes of the person they are caring for with this disease, setting them up for an impactful connection. An impactful connection leads to successful care.

Soon after using this model with my patients, I was teaching others to use it, and they found great success with their patients and loved ones. Their feedback—how they wished they had learned this years earlier and how it truly helped them understand and move forward with effective strategies—kept my motivation to continue to teach others and even to write this book to reach a larger audience.

The three prongs of the Dementia Connection Model are known in the health care industry, but this is the first time they have been put into practice together. The origin of the model, and first prong, is based on the theory of retrogenesis, that as dementia progresses, the individual's skills, experiences, and memories all go in reverse to birth. The research backing this theory finds that people experiencing the moderate to late stages of the disease have a developmental age of 7 years to 4 weeks old. Children in this age range experience the world differently compared to adults and learn through their senses rather than relying on factual knowledge, which helps explain why individuals with a progressed form of the disease experience their world differently than those around them. The second prong, habilitation, focuses on the abilities of those living with dementia rather than on their disabilities. We know that people with dementia can still feel emotions because we observe their mood changes early on in the disease; we also know that they will experience their world, both learning and engagement, using their senses more and more as the disease progresses. We will use these two nuggets to our advantage for connecting to our patients and loved ones. Lastly comes the intervention. The third prong is called sensory-based knowledge and information. We will use sensory stimulation methods to influence our patient's or loved one's feelings in a positive way, similar to the approach we use with children, because they are taking in that sensory-based information through their senses to understand it. If the individual feels happy, safe, secure, and loved, they will connect more to the person providing this positive stimulation. Furthermore, if the person is positively reinforced each time, the likelihood that they will continue the positive behavior increases. On the other side, the person caring for them feels successful, confident, and at peace that their patient or loved one is happy and comfortable. It's a win-win!

This book is intentionally set up in a workbook style so that you can learn about this model and how it applies to common symptoms of dementia, allowing you to compare the symptoms your loved one is experiencing. Then, you'll use the Dementia Connection Model with your loved one to see what works for them, journaling what was successful and building a toolbox of interventions to use.

This work reviews the basics about what dementia is and the common symptoms it involves. Unlike other books about dementia, however, this one goes into greater depth regarding why individuals with dementia experience their world differently than you and I and why they have the particular symptoms that go along with the disease. It then teaches you the hands-on approaches you can use every day. Not only will your loved one feel positive emotions when you are using this model, but you will feel positive as well.

Although this book does not cover the various forms of dementia, I have found that this model can very much be transferable when caring for those with other types. Just try it.

If this book ends up being all you need, then keep this book and your notes around for whenever you might need them. But if you are in the pursuit of more information, feel free to check out my website, NeuroEssence, at neuroessence.org. Also, the Alzheimer's Association (alz.org) has useful and engaging tools for families and caregivers. They provide information, guidance, and resources that can help build upon what you've learned here. I encourage you to read a great deal about this disease, as we continuously research and learn more about it. We still need a cure.

Acknowledgments

The journey of writing this book and putting my ideas and interventions into thoughts, instruction, and ultimately a model to use and follow would not have been possible without the support of a number of influential people in my life.

I first thank Mary Beth Janssen for encouraging me to write my first book. She inspired me to pursue my dreams by what she's done in her career and the books she has written, not leaving it to someone else to spread the word. I probably wouldn't have taken that leap of faith without her telling me, "You were meant to do this." I so vividly remember that phone call.

I'd like to give a very special thanks to my husband, Jack. When I was discouraged after several publisher proposal submissions with no bites, he personally sat down and looked up more for me. He pinpointed Johns Hopkins University Press (JHUP). If it wasn't for his belief in me, my dreams, and this book, then this may not have been possible. I also thank him for all his love and support as we navigated this journey together. I spent many hours writing, and he kept encouraging me to write more, as he took on primary responsibilities with our little ones and taking care of the house at times. I know it wasn't easy when he felt like he was doing it all. One of the many reasons I fell in love with him is because of his positivity and quest to be in the moment—qualities that have helped me in my writing.

I'd like to thank Rachael Wonderlin, an author who has published with JHUP and an accomplished dementia care leader, for her incredible editing skills, guidance and support, words of encouragement, honesty, and experience. Although

I felt moments of frustration and defeat while on this journey, she helped me to "just write" and not overthink it. I was able to finally feel what she meant. She truly is an inspiration for entrepreneurs.

Many thanks to JHUP, especially to Joe Rusko and his team, for giving me this opportunity to share my knowledge, passion, and approach to dementia care with so many and to fulfill one of my lifelong dreams.

I am grateful to all the clinical researchers, clinicians, and professionals who developed the concepts discussed in this model. They are integral in the treatment of those living with dementia.

I also appreciate my family, friends, and colleagues for the faith I felt backing me. Their love and support were with me at every step. I dedicated this book to my children—Jackson, now age 6, and Julianna, now age 4. Watching and studying their every move since they were babies, as I was taking care of those who have dementia, made the idea, concepts, and interventions come alive. I personally want to thank my sister, Mickey, for opening the door to the forward-thinking approach of an inspirational guru who helped me view things differently and encourages everyone to strive for more. My sister was my cheerleader, often checking in and celebrating with me at each milestone of this journey. I also want to thank my mother, as I can always see in her eyes how proud she is of me throughout my life and during this pursuit. I know my father is looking down from above with that same sentiment. The two of them have showed me what a good work ethic is and taught me that if you work hard, your dreams will come true.

I want to also thank the Alden Network, including my directors and their teams, for humoring me about the million and one ideas I've had over the years and for their contribution to making this model possible with their thoughts, ideas, and willingness to put it into action, proving its success. And last, but not least, another thank-you is needed for my business partner at NeuroEssence, Jessica, for believing in my work and continuing to generate excitement around potential business opportunities for our mission.

A special acknowledgment goes to my grandfather, who is my inspiration for brain health. My papa lived a good, long life, he'd say. Papa wanted to make it until this book was published, and to surpass his 100th birthday; however, he decided it was time when he was 99. I know how proud of me he was. He was honored to be my muse for this pursuit. I will forever be thankful. I know he will read this from above. Rest in peace, Papa.

The Busy Caregiver's Guide to
Advanced Alzheimer Disease

What Is Alzheimer Disease?

There is more than one answer to the question, "What is Alzheimer disease?" From people who have Alzheimer disease to health care professionals who treat them to loved ones who care for them, the answers to this question will be slightly different. But from the different answers emerges a common pattern that describes the general experience of Alzheimer disease—what health care professionals call the "clinical picture." In this book, I focus on that clinical picture—what happens during the journey of Alzheimer disease, both for those who have it and those who care for them. My hope is that you will understand the "why?" of this disease: "Why does my loved one act like this? Why can't they do this anymore? Why do they say these things? Why can't they understand what I'm saying or asking them to do?" Understanding the "why?" gives you a base to start. Then, I will introduce and share a cognitive-behavioral approach to care called the Dementia Connection Model, which ties together three key concepts in our understanding of the clinical picture of Alzheimer's. I hope this model will help you better understand some of what is happening to your loved one—and to *you*—on your caregiving journey.

Another set of answers to the question "What is Alzheimer disease?" relates to what causes Alzheimer disease and whether it can be prevented, cured, or slowed down. After decades of research and much progress, the unfortunate truth is that we still don't know all the details of those answers. In this chapter, I share the current understanding and theories from researchers that inform the three key concepts of the Dementia Connection Model—retrogenesis, habilitation, and sensory-based knowledge—to help you better understand how and why the Dementia Connection Model works.

THE BASICS

Whether this is the first book you are reading about Alzheimer disease or the next of many books you have learned from, I hope to provide an understanding of the disease or to expand it, specifically with respect to the Dementia Connection Model. Bear with me on the more technical clinical information, but it's necessary to understand the full picture of Alzheimer disease.

Alzheimer disease is defined as a neurocognitive disorder in the American Psychiatric Association's *Diagnostic and Statistical Manual of Mental Disorders*, now in its 5th edition, and as a neurodegenerative disease in the 10th edition of *International Classification of Disease*. The disease was first discovered by Dr. Alois Alzheimer, a clinical psychiatrist and neuroanatomist. In 1906, Dr. Alzheimer found during an autopsy that there were changes in the brain of a woman he had treated for five years; she had had paranoia, sleep disturbances, aggression, confusion, and memory deficits. Dr. Alzheimer noted that her brain had distinctive plaques and neurofibrillary tangles. Between 1909 and 1911, he found similar brain changes on autopsies of three other individuals who had had similar symptoms. As was common for neurologic and psychiatric diseases at the time, these findings were named after the physician who discovered them, and in 1910, the term *Alzheimer's disease* was first used in print.[1]

For some time after the early twentieth century, a practitioner could not give someone a diagnosis of Alzheimer disease until the person had died and an autopsy showed the same plaques and tangles that Dr. Alzheimer first identified in 1906. Today, a practitioner can diagnose Alzheimer disease or one of its variants with 90% certainty while an individual is still living. But there is no *single* test that can determine whether a person has Alzheimer disease. Several tests by different professionals—neurologists and neuropsychologists, primarily—are needed to make a firm diagnosis of Alzheimer disease. New methods for imaging, or taking pictures of, the brain, and proteins within it, are being developed to help diagnose Alzheimer disease more accurately, but so far these methods are rarely used outside of research because their true accuracy isn't yet well understood.[2]

Some researchers are investigating whether measuring the amount of those same proteins in the blood or fluid from inside the spinal column (cerebrospinal fluid) could be used to diagnose Alzheimer disease. This type of test cannot currently be performed outside of a research lab, however.[3] Gene testing is a promising new tool, as several research outcomes point to about ten genes that may indicate that a person is predisposed to dementia; the *APOE* genes are the ones closely associated with Alzheimer disease.

The plaques and tangles that Alois Alzheimer discovered have contributed much to what we know about how Alzheimer disease affects the brain and to tests that are being developed.[4,5] Imaging and fluid tests measure the proteins found in the plaques and tangles that are the hallmark of Alzheimer disease. Plaques are made mostly of amyloid (*am-uh-loyd*), and beta-amyloid 42 specifically is one form that is thought to be especially toxic. When abnormal levels of beta-amyloid 42 are formed, the protein clumps together (or aggregates) outside of cells, forming a plaque that is thought to disrupt connections between nerve cells.

Like muscles, nerve cells depend on one another for activity. Without activity, nerve cells die and degenerate. This leads the brain to deteriorate over time, causing further brain cell death and shrinkage (also called atrophy). It's much like how termites eat away at wood; little by little, the wood is gone. As the brain shrinks, less of the neurotransmitter acetylcholine (*uh-see-tul-ko-lean*) is produced, which further affects the overall balance of neurotransmitters and signaling between nerve cells. Eventually, the left and right hemispheres aren't able to communicate with each other. The neurofibrillary (fibrous) tangles that Dr. Alzheimer observed also form within cells near the amyloid plaques and are seen as the sites of brain shrinkage. These tangles are accumulations of the protein tau (rhymes with *how*), a protein that is used within nerve cells to transport substances outside the body of the cells in the brain. In Alzheimer disease, tau disrupts the process of communication between cells.

There has been much research on the possible causes of the plaques and tangles, but researchers still don't know exactly what causes them. The amyloid hypothesis suggests that buildup of abnormal amyloid triggers the whole process of plaque and tangle formation and brain atrophy. The tau hypothesis suggests that buildup of tau in addition to beta-amyloid is what triggers the disease. Recently, many investi-

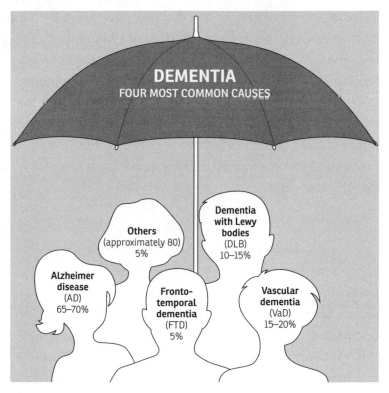

Types of dementia

gational potential drugs aimed at lowering beta-amyloid levels have failed to improve the symptoms of Alzheimer disease in clinical trials. As a result, the amyloid hypothesis has been called into question, and additional research has been done into other potential causes. But the amyloid hypothesis has not been disproven because there are many reasons that these trials may have failed.[6] In addition to studying amyloid and tau, researchers are studying the role that sleep, diet, and exercise may have in protecting the brain from Alzheimer disease and the role that exposure to certain infections, metals, or pesticides may have in making Alzheimer disease more likely.[7,8]

Dementia is not defined as a disease or diagnosis. Dementia is an umbrella term for a collection of symptoms, including problems in memory, language, orientation (knowing when and where you are), learning ability, and judgment. Depending on what is causing dementia, an individual may experience all of these symptoms or just a few. More than one hundred causes of dementia have been discovered. Alzheimer disease is the most common cause of dementia; it accounts for two-thirds of cases.

THE SIZE OF THE PROBLEM

In case you have not been told yet or haven't heard it recently—*you are not alone.* As I write this book in 2020, there are approximately 5 million Americans who have Alzheimer disease. It is estimated that by 2050, more than 16 million Americans will have it. Someone develops Alzheimer disease every 66 seconds.[5]

Alzheimer disease is the most common new diagnosis for people 65 or older and is the fifth-leading cause of death for people in that age group. Although rare, what is called "early onset" or "younger onset" Alzheimer disease can occur in people between the ages of 30 and 50.

Alzheimer disease is more common in women than in men. This is simply because age makes Alzheimer disease more likely, and women live longer. Another reason may result from differences in female biology, a topic of debate and ongoing research.[5]

African Americans and Hispanics are 2 and 1.5 times, respectively, more likely to develop Alzheimer disease than whites. The reasons for this disparity are also not well understood. Some studies suggest the increase in Alzheimer disease among African Americans and Hispanics may be linked to greater rates of diabetes, high cholesterol, and cardiovascular disease in these communities. Other studies are investigating whether there are biological differences in these groups; this can be difficult to determine because in most research studies to date, the majority of participants have been white.[5]

Of the top-ten causes of death, Alzheimer disease is the only one without a cure. Many research organizations and advocacy groups are trying to change this. There has also been a shift in research focus to understand whether it might be possible to slow down or even prevent Alzheimer disease through lifestyle changes that promote brain health.[7,8]

THE CLINICAL PICTURE CHANGES WITH TIME

Mild Cognitive Impairment

Many people who eventually develop Alzheimer disease first had mild cognitive impairment (MCI). In MCI, a person and their close family and friends might notice they are forgetful or have trouble thinking, but it is not severe enough to keep them from doing everyday activities. Not everyone who develops MCI will go on to have Alzheimer disease. In fact, only 15% to 20% of people age 65 and older have MCI, and merely 15% of people with MCI develop Alzheimer disease annually. Statistically, that means that in a group of 100 seniors, 20 would have MCI, but only 3 would go on to develop Alzheimer disease at some point within a year.

A person with MCI may experience subtle difficulties with cognitive issues, like planning, organizing, and forgetfulness. People with MCI may be unable to remember names of people who were just introduced. They may frequently forget where they parked their car or put their keys. Additionally, they might not be able to recall conversations they had, or they tell individuals in their lives the same story repeatedly, even after being informed they've told that story before. Others might start to notice these types of lapses, including the individual themselves.

It is important to remember that occasional memory lapses happen to everyone at any age and that they do occur more frequently with normal aging. Forgetting where you put your keys now and then and being able to find them on your own is not MCI. Forgetting them regularly and always needing help to find them may suggest an evaluation is needed. Remember that roughly 80% of those age 65 and older do not develop MCI each year, and 85% of people who have MCI won't develop Alzheimer disease. Additionally, research is showing that there are things we can all do to protect our brain health and possibly lower our risk for Alzheimer disease.[6,7] Because many people who care for those with Alzheimer disease fear that they will eventually develop it too, I have included a bonus chapter at the end of this book that summarizes the latest research on keeping your brain healthy. Research indicates these techniques are helpful even for those who already have MCI or early Alzheimer disease (see chapter 14, "Promoting Brain Health").

Mr. Stewart Was Going to Whose Wedding?

After I wrapped up a community training seminar on dementia care, an attendee, Mr. Stewart, came up to me. With concern on his face, he told me about a recent conversation he'd had with his son Dan, who had been preparing for his wedding—scheduled for the next weekend—for quite some time. As they were talking, Dan asked his dad about plans for the upcoming weekend, thinking outside of any plans related to the wedding. When Mr. Stewart replied that he was going to a wedding, Dan looked at him oddly and said, "Dad, it's my wedding you are going to." Mr. Stewart confessed, "Doc, I was so embarrassed." He admitted struggling with memory issues for some time, but knowing that his son now noticed was really a wakeup call for him. We discussed the next steps he could take, and he seemed to feel at ease having direction.

Early Alzheimer Disease

As discussed above, Alzheimer disease causes brain atrophy. One of the first areas where this occurs is in the medial temporal lobe, which is responsible for understanding time and navigation. The medial temporal lobe, or entorhinal (*en-toe-rye-nal*) cortex, also connects the limbic system, where memory and emotion reside, to the neocortex and frontal lobe, which is responsible for executive functions like planning, organizing, problem solving, anticipating risks, and having self-control. Atrophy progresses, or spreads, from the entorhinal cortex to the limbic system, especially the hippocampus, which is responsible for memory, and the amygdala, which regulates mood and emotion. The frontal lobe will eventually atrophy as well.[9]

Understanding this pattern of atrophy helps us to understand how symptoms progress and change over time with Alzheimer disease. Early on, an individual will experience forgetfulness, concentration difficulties, and short-term memory loss, like knowing how to get home or remembering to pay bills, go to appointments, or take medication. Personality and mood will start to change, and people may not seem like themselves. They may then struggle with independent skills, such as managing money, driving safely, traveling to new places, planning parties or get-togethers, organizing schedules, and

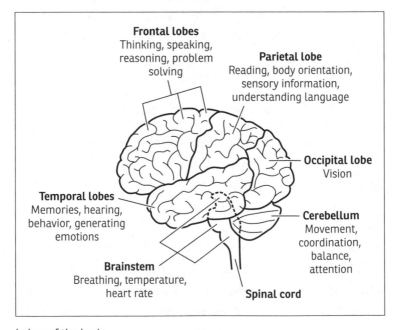

Lobes of the brain

creating appointment times. Eventually, speech and language begin to become a struggle, like trying to find words and coordinating mouth and speech movements.

Later in the early stages, an individual may start to forget names of family members, usually first with grandchildren then children (not yet who they are but their names). Judgment begins to be affected, and the basic activities of grooming and self-care may become problematic.

Although the pattern of progressive atrophy and related symptoms described here is most typical, atrophy does not follow the same pattern in every individual. Different people may have symptoms occur in different orders and may not have every symptom described here.

Moderate-Stage Alzheimer Disease

In the middle stage of Alzheimer disease, the atrophy of the frontal lobe and problems with executive function worsen. An individual will require some supervision because safety issues become more evident. Typically at this stage, family members start to look for a safe, supervised place where their loved one can live and be cared for. Other brain areas that are involved in speech, hearing, and vision are also likely to be affected. Two types of language problems occur. One is having difficulty finding the words to express something, and the other is having difficulty naming objects, which eventually develops into not understanding an object's function. For example, an individual with Alzheimer's will know what a fork does for quite a while in the disease process but will forget that it is called a fork. Eventually, they will lose the understanding or purpose of a fork.

Eyesight may worsen, which can cause problems with depth perception and peripheral vision, including not being able to distinguish lighter colors, having the illusion that darker colors below the knees look like holes in the ground, or not being able to see on the sides or above or below the vision area.

Mood may continue to change to more of a negative state over time, and mood swings may become more common.

When the parietal (*pah-rye-et-tal*) area—the middle and top part of the brain—is affected, it becomes difficult for the individual to know where things are around them or even where their own limbs are in relation to their body. For example, an individual with moderate Alzheimer disease will have difficulty touching their nose with their finger without looking at their finger (a common exercise that can be used in the diagnostic procedures). Additionally, they might not know where the edge of the bed, seat, or toilet is or where the end of the wall, countertop, or door is. In combination with problems in areas of the brain that control movement, parietal problems lead to bumps, frequent trips and falls, and limited walking and mobility.

As Alzheimer disease continues to worsen, difficulty with time can lead to confusing the different parts of the day. Short-term memory may be completely absent, and long-term memory becomes affected. A person with this stage of Alzheimer disease struggles to remember events of their own life. Typically, more recent events are forgotten before earlier events, so grandchildren are likely to be forgotten before children, who may be forgotten before a spouse. Children are sometimes perceived as siblings, and people with Alzheimer disease refer to times when they were teenagers and children as though they are happening now. In contrast, events that occur after those memories may be completely lost.

It is common for people at this stage to nap during the day and progressively stay awake at night. Eating habits also will change, with people usually favoring sweeter foods.

Toward the end of this phase, more and more supervision will be needed. Urinary and/or fecal incontinence may occur. People can develop fixed false beliefs, see or hear things that are not there, or have obsessions, usually all relating to past memories. Anxiety and fear, and possibly aggression, may occur.

Advanced Alzheimer Disease

In the final phases of Alzheimer disease, the entire brain is affected and most to all independent and basic life skills are lost. At this stage, an individual with Alzheimer disease will need supervision 24 hours a day, 7 days a week and total assistance with care. People with advanced Alzheimer disease may not be able to leave their beds and are likely not to remember their family and friends. The ability to speak is often limited to the use of single, intelligible words that may be repeated over and over. A person may not be able to show emotions through facial expressions and will likely experience difficulty chewing and swallowing, limited to no motor coordination, and bowel and bladder incontinence.

THE UNVEILING

The amygdala is part of the limbic system, which typically atrophies early in the disease. The amygdala is responsible primarily for processing and remembering emotional reactions and triggering our fight-or-flight response (our innate coping skills). As atrophy occurs, the ability to *regulate* and *control* emotional responses becomes impaired. Commonly, psychological symptoms are present before there are functional deficits. Eventually, approximately 80% of people with Alzheimer's have psychological symptoms, including anxiety, agitation, mood dysregulation, paranoia, thought disturbances, and seeing or hearing things that aren't present. These psychological symptoms and other evidence suggest people with Alzheimer disease can still feel emotions for a very long time. Toward the middle to end of Alzheimer disease, a person may not be able to express how they feel in words or with facial expressions but may still have a full range of emotions. Additionally, our innate fight-or-flight response as self-protection may become more likely. It is helpful to keep this unveiling information at the front of your mind as you continue to read this book and care for your loved one with Alzheimer disease. More to come in chapter 2.

SUMMARY

Although there is a common pattern of symptoms and changes over time that most people with Alzheimer disease will follow during their journey, the progression won't be exactly the same for every individual. What research has shown so far is that

Alzheimer disease is related to a toxic buildup of proteins that leads to a sequence of degeneration and atrophy (shrinking) of specific areas of the brain. The sequence of where atrophy happens helps us to understand how the symptoms, or clinical picture, of Alzheimer disease changes over time. In the next chapter, I explain how the clinical picture helps us understand the three key components of the Dementia Connection Model: retrogenesis, habilitation, and sensory-based knowledge.

What Is the Dementia Connection Model?

The Dementia Connection Model brings together three concepts in dementia care that help caregivers understand what is happening to the person with Alzheimer disease and, more importantly, what our loved ones need as their condition progresses and how to successfully intervene. It's a road map that helps connect you and your loved one in a way that produces positive interactions and preserves your loved one's level of functioning for as long as possible. The Dementia Connection Model is a cognitive-behavioral technique in the dementia care world, if you will.

RETROGENESIS

The first concept in the Dementia Connection Model is the theory of *retrogenesis*, which was developed by Dr. Barry Reisberg.[1] The theory of retrogenesis says a person with Alzheimer disease loses brain functions in the reverse order that they learned them. How we feed ourselves serves as a useful example. When we were infants, we drank milk from a bottle or breast using a reflex that we didn't even have to learn. Later, we learned to hold the bottle. Then we could sit up and were fed baby food of a soft consistency, and we tried new foods. Eventually, as we developed the ability to grasp objects with a thumb and forefinger, we could bring small pieces of food to our mouths. We started to eat off a spoon that was held for us, and eventually we grabbed the spoon and started to learn how to use utensils to feed ourselves independently by watching others. Gradually, we learned to drink from cups instead of bottles, first with lids and then with open cups and glasses.

Mary's Mother Eats Like Mary's Granddaughter

Mary said that her mother, Joyce, typically used her fork and spoon without a problem. Then, slowly over time, she noticed that her mother would hold her fork in her hand while using her free hand to bring food to her mouth. Mary didn't understand why her mother kept doing this. "I encourage her to use her utensils. At times I even find myself getting frustrated with her," Mary explained. Despite her daughter's insistence that she use utensils, Joyce continued to eat with her hands. Mary found this interesting because her first granddaughter, only a year old, was eating in a similar way. She saw her granddaughter eat food with her hands, and then later eat using one hand and one fork.

When Joyce came into our care, Mary asked us if her mother's inability to use utensils was a "normal" progression of the disease and whether there was any relationship between her mother and granddaughter's similar way of eating.

This learning process reverses for a person with Alzheimer disease. With eating, this means that they may first need adaptable equipment—like a cup with a lid—to prevent any spilling while drinking or thicker utensils that are easier to grasp. The ability to use utensils will eventually be lost, and a person will eat with their fingers once the meaning of what utensils are used for is lost. Then, people with Alzheimer's will need to transition over time from regular food to precut small bites to softer foods to assist with swallowing and prevent choking. Eventually, in the late stages of disease, it will be necessary for them to be fed by their caregivers. In this manner, the individual's journey goes in reverse of how an infant learns to eat. This is what is meant by retrogenesis, or in other words, retrogression or regression.

Another realm affected by retrogenesis is language. When infants are born, they cry to get their needs met. They move on from crying to cooing and babbling, quickly learning language sounds. Soon, they say their first words, and later they learn more words and put them together. They eventually speak in short sentences and then in longer ones. An individual with Alzheimer disease experiences this in reverse as the disease progresses, first with shorter sentences and then a few words. They will progress to using only one or two words, and eventually the person can communicate verbally only by crying out.

Mobility, too, is affected in this way. When infants are born, they are placed on their back or belly, but they do not know how to roll over. Eventually they learn how to roll over, sit up, crawl, pull up, walk with the aid of toys or by holding onto furniture, and then walk independently. Again, retrogenesis tells us this will occur in reverse in a person with Alzheimer disease. We see that our loved one with Alzheimer's may first need to hold a cane to walk, then a walker, eventually progressing to a wheelchair. They finally may reach the point when it is difficult to sit up and roll over. At that stage, a person with Alzheimer disease may spend a lot of time reclining in a chair or lying in bed.

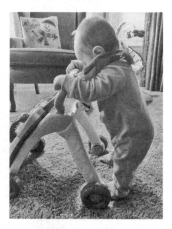

Infant walking with the aid of a toy

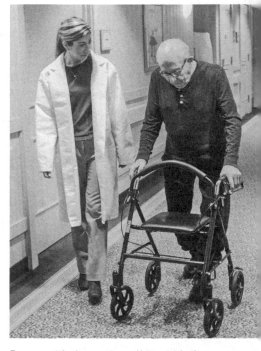

Person with dementia walking with the assistance of a walker and a guide

Reisberg's research shows that someone with late-stage Alzheimer disease may have a mental age of anywhere from 7 years to 4 weeks old. Not only is their brain weight comparable, but the general skill set and abilities of someone with late-stage dementia are similar to a very young child. Just as we notice young people starting to (sometimes!) behave as adults in their late teens, caregivers start to notice changes in their loved one with Alzheimer disease when their developmental level has regressed to that of a teenager. There is a silver lining: you will possibly get to know what your loved one was like at an earlier time in their lives and share those earlier likes, dislikes, and personality with them. In the midst of this devastating disease, this takeaway is pretty cool.

Retrogenesis reminds us that it is vital for care partners to accept that the developmental age of their loved one will eventually not match their chronological age. To clarify, Reisberg's literature does not say to treat people with Alzheimer disease like children. What it does tell us is that we can use the knowledge of what young children are capable of and some of the same strategies and techniques that are successful with younger people to interact, communicate, and connect in a meaningful and productive way. The Dementia Connection Model uses a dignified approach, as detailed in the intervention chapters later in the book.

The significance of this information is crucial when caring for and connecting with your loved one. Many caregivers feel as though they are on a hamster wheel—running around and around, repeating the same interactions over and over—with no or limited successful impact on the actions of their loved one, no matter what they do. This can leave caregivers feeling understandably confused, frustrated, and hopeless. Understanding retrogenesis puts things in perspective. Knowing that the person you care for is functioning like someone at a younger age leads to a better understanding of what they can or can't do. This understanding allows you, as a caregiver, to have more realistic expectations that hopefully bring greater acceptance of what you and your loved one are experiencing. Once care partners accept that retrogression is occurring in their loved ones, caregiving gets a lot easier. It becomes easier to let go of expectations and focus on the positive aspects of taking care of and spending time with the person you love.

Retrogenesis Explains the Connection between Mary's Mother and Granddaughter

Mary felt frustrated because she kept telling Joyce to use her utensils day after day, to no avail. But it was not that Joyce didn't want to cooperate with her daughter's requests, she just could not understand how to use utensils as her dementia progressed. Joyce eventually ate with her hands, adapting to her new world and abilities to maintain independence while eating. Mary had to learn to accept her mother's new world, even if that world was similar to her granddaughter's.

HABILITATION

Mary's experience with her mother is more common than not for many caregivers. Her attention was focused on what her mother, Joyce, could not do for herself anymore, which led to much frustration for Mary. What if we turn this thought process around? What if, instead of focusing on and getting frustrated about what individuals with Alzheimer disease cannot do anymore, we shift our focus to what they *can* do. This requires a "glass half full" mentality to focus on a person's remaining abilities and reinforce those that may help them keep some skills longer than they would have otherwise. This idea—*habilitation*—is the second concept of the Dementia Connection Model, focusing on an individual's abilities and reinforcing and using them daily to maintain them for as long as possible.

Joyce was using the skills that she still had; bringing food to her mouth with her hands was important so that she could maintain some independence. Although the theory of retrogenesis indicates that people with advanced Alzheimer disease are developmentally moving toward a younger age, there are skills and abilities they can still use.

How do we know what abilities those living with Alzheimer disease still have? As the disease progresses, someone with advanced Alzheimer disease will not be able to learn new things *related to factual knowledge*. This is because the area of the brain responsible for generating new fact-based memories—the hippocampus—is shrinking, as discussed in chapter 1. People with dementia can still learn; however, they learn the way a younger person does, through repetition and experience, utilizing the information that is picked up through their senses. After all, an infant learning to use a cup doesn't read a manual telling them what the function of the cup handle is. They watch, listen, and try repeatedly. Then they learn, using the information from their senses to make sense of their world and how to navigate in it. Those with moderate to progressed dementia will use this same way of learning to adapt. You probably have heard that people with dementia experience the world differently than you and I; this is what that means.

Procedural memory is an unconscious long-term memory process that assists with the performance of particular tasks without awareness.[2] An example is riding a bicycle. Once you know how, you just get on and do it without thinking through all the steps that you once had to learn. Skills saved in procedural memory are automatically retrieved and executed without any conscious effort. Procedural memory is created through procedural learning, which means repeating a complex activity over and over again until it can be done without consciously thinking about it. Individuals with progressing Alzheimer disease will still struggle with and lose these abilities over time, but habilitation—if the decline is observed early enough and the skills are reinforced—may help them keep some skills for a longer time. Research has shown that individuals with Alzheimer disease have abilities—and may be able to regain some abilities—when provided the habilitation to do so.[2] Care providers who focus on these abilities and reinforce them may see the most success.

Also, in chapter 1, I unveiled that emotions are present even if not expressed—and that lost control over emotions and atrophy of the amygdala mean more mood swings and more negative emotions coming to the surface. Some people living with dementia may not be able to tell others how they are feeling anymore, because they are slowly losing their language abilities and may not be able to show their feelings through facial expressions as readily. But we know they still can feel emotions because we observe their negative emotions through their body language, or what is called behaviors. Caregivers can use this knowledge to make things better for the cared-for person and even themselves by changing negative emotions into positive ones.

If you could choose the emotions your loved one with Alzheimer disease felt, which would they be? Which do you wish they could experience for the rest of their life? You would opt for positive emotions of security, safety, calm, joy, and happiness. Right?

SENSORY-BASED KNOWLEDGE

Our emotions are influenced through our senses. What we see, hear, taste, smell, and touch influences how we feel. Music, for example, is a form of auditory (hearing) stimulation. Listening to upbeat, "feel-good" music makes us feel positive and energetic. In contrast, sad, dreary music can cause us to feel lackluster and distraught. Similar feelings can be aroused by food. We may reminisce when the taste of what we are eating reminds us of something, either positive or negative. Our feelings will be influenced based on how we felt in that moment. Stimuli coming through our senses influences our emotions. The third concept in the Dementia Connection Model is *sensory-based knowledge*, which makes use of this connection between our senses and our feelings.

Going back to the first and second concepts of the Dementia Connection Model, retrogenesis tells us that people with Alzheimer disease are developmentally getting younger, experiencing the world differently than you and I—similarly to young people—and habilitation tells us they can continue learning with procedural memory. Senses and feelings inform that learning—just as was true when we were all infants. As we reached for something, feeling it with a hand and grasping it—perhaps a parent clapped or gave praise when we did—the sense of touch and positive feelings drove our learning to use the cup. Senses and feelings can also be used to help the person with Alzheimer disease and you, their care partner. In order to learn procedurally, a person with Alzheimer disease will have to rely heavily on sensory-based, not fact-based, knowledge.

As a caregiver, you can connect better by intentionally creating and using constructive affirmative stimulation daily to influence emotions positively, which encourages learning and maintenance of skills. This is the exact way infants and children learn before the age of 5.

The Dementia Connection Model in Practice

Betty was having a particularly tough afternoon. As the hours wore on, she started to become agitated with the people around her. She was wandering with an angry look, cursing, unwilling to listen, and trying to push people away if they became physically close. Betty repeated to herself, "I want to go home; I want to go home."

I stepped in to help calm Betty and prevent any further escalation. Approaching Betty gently, I presented myself in a calm manner with a smile on my face. I spoke to Betty in a calm, monotone voice. I played soothing sounds, used a lavender essential oil blend, and gave her a light touch so she knew that she was safe. Betty calmed down within minutes and even wanted to spend more time together.

Through the Dementia Connection Model, I knew that Betty could still feel emotions, even positive ones if influenced effectively (habilitation). I knew she experienced her world differently than I did by taking information in through her senses (sensory-based information), like young ones do (retrogenesis). So I used affirmative stimuli to provide auditory, olfactory, and tactile stimulation to influence a sense of calm. Appealing to Betty's senses helped to deescalate the moment, which made me feel calm and confident for helping her. In the future, Betty will likely continue to feel a sense of peace when she sees me, because she has learned to attribute that positive feeling and behavior with me. She's calm, I'm calm.

THE DEMENTIA CONNECTION MODEL

The three pillars of the Dementia Connection Model tell us that people with Alzheimer disease are developmentally younger than their real age and learn with sensory-based procedural learning. This is an old-new world for them—watching, listening, mimicking, and learning through their senses. Through this process, they can also remember how they feel about people. Names and roles may not be recalled, but the feelings stick. It's important that every interaction is accompanied by a positive mood and interaction. Pay attention to your nonverbal language, such as facial expressions and body language. Pay attention to what sense you are stimulating. Pay attention to what works, to what makes them happy.

To implement the Dementia Connection Model, use the three R's—routine, remind, reward.[3] If the caregiver consistently (routine) provides sensory cues (remind), then the cared-for person and the caregiver will be happy (reward). This is the best recipe for a win-win!

Knowing this information, care partners can emotionally and physically connect with their loved ones with Alzheimer disease by positively influencing their senses through the use of affirmative sensory stimulation. Caregivers can help change negative thoughts, emotions, and behaviors into positive thoughts, emotions, and behaviors. Interactions should be intentional, meaning you try to influence positive emotions by creating, targeting, and using affirmative sensory experiences for what will be seen, heard, tasted, smelled, and touched. Intentional interactions are a more productive and meaningful way to connect to your loved one to help influence feelings of safety, security, and happiness. You will quickly realize that you have found a way into their new world, which will leave you feeling successful, confident, and accomplished. Win-win!

Using the Dementia Connection Model

There are several affirmative stimuli that you can use to influence someone's emotions in a positive way. In this chapter, I introduce a few stimuli that can be especially helpful when caring for a person with Alzheimer disease. How and when these can best be used are discussed in future chapters.

STIMULATING SIGHT

Nonverbal Communication

Nonverbal communication is visual stimulation that can say a lot to a person without saying anything at all. People living with dementia respond well when the people around them appear to be in a happy mood, much like young people do when they are around adults. Consider the old sales tip to smile when talking on the phone, because the smile lights up your face and projects through your voice, also influencing verbal communication. Nonverbal happiness appears as a smile, relaxed shoulders and arms, direct eye contact, and slow, steady movements. When you are interacting and communicating with the person you care for, pay attention to what your nonverbal communication is saying. Whenever possible, you want to show a positive, happy mood.

In chapter 2, I discussed how individuals with dementia, like young children, mimic others as part of procedural skills-based learning. Picture this: a toddler is running down the sidewalk. She's running to her heart's content, giggling and smiling. All the while, though, her mom is thinking, "Gosh, I hope she doesn't fall." The little girl keeps running, and there she goes . . . to the ground . . . skidding on her knees and palms. Her first reaction is to turn around to look at mom, to gauge mom's reaction, so she knows how to react. Mom has two options here. She can either show a look of panic and gasp out of fear and hurt for her little baby, or she can show a look of hope, admiration, and smiles indicating that all will be ok. The second option will keep her daughter calm and the situation lighthearted. Daughter is happy; mom is happy. Win-win!

People with Alzheimer disease often mimic another person's mood. If you are having a bad day, you may need to "fake it until you make it." A positive mood sets the tone for any interaction or communication, leading to a meaningful connection. You know the saying, "First impressions count." Well, first impressions count every time with an individual who has dementia. This will set you up for success. I discuss more on communication in chapter 4.

Art

Studies show that art can be a beneficial therapeutic technique for adults, specifically for individuals with dementia.[1] It's an outlet to release emotions on paper when a person can no longer find the words to express themselves verbally. Art is a form of tactile and visual stimulation. According to the Alzheimer's Association website,[2] "Art projects can create a sense of accomplishment and purpose. They can provide the person with dementia—as well as caregivers—an opportunity for self-expression." The theory of retrogenesis tells us that coloring and drawing are forms of expression for people with Alzheimer disease, just as they are for toddlers and young children. Focusing on simple tasks, like coloring, also helps to relieve anxiety and stress. All forms of art—coloring, drawing, or making crafts—help children and older people alike express themselves. It's best to ensure that any pictures, utensils, or products are items that adults would use but are nontoxic in case they are ingested.

Colors

Color is another visual stimulus that can influence mood. Many colors are associated with emotions like "seeing red" or "feeling blue," although these associations are not always consistent from one culture to another.[3]

Red is an attention-getting color. Dinner plates in many dementia care settings are red, as the color was found to increase food consumption in people with Alzheimer disease.[4] The contrast between the food and the red plate helps patients see the food better. Red can also be used to draw people out; painting the inside of a door red may incite a person to leave their room.[5] Red shoes may promote going for a walk, red cups may encourage drinking, a red ball may prompt participation in a game, and so on. As an attention-getting color, however, red can also be distracting or threatening and is not the best choice for clothing when you are caring for someone with dementia.

Blue is known to be a calming color. A room that is painted blue may reduce confusion and increase concentration.[4] Blue light has been shown to lower heart rate and blood pressure. But too much blue light can interfere with sleep, so the American Academy of Sleep Medicine recommends limiting blue light during the 30 minutes before bedtime.

Green often symbolizes growth and life, and can also be calming and attention-getting. The human eye is most sensitive to green light; green is often the last color a person can differentiate.

STIMULATING HEARING

Verbal Communication

Just as with nonverbal communication, the person with Alzheimer disease for whom you are caring will notice your overall demeanor. As your mother might have said, "It's not what you say, it's how you say it," and that is true in caring for those with dementia. Your tone, cadence, and volume are important pieces of verbal communication. A calm and gentle voice is a pleasant form of auditory (related to hearing) stimulation. When a cared-for person hears a reassuring voice, they are likely to mimic it, increasing the likelihood of a calm demeanor in your loved one. More to come in chapter 4.

Music

Music is a powerful auditory stimulus that can influence mood, making people feel happy, sad, angry, nostalgic, and so much more. Music taps into our limbic system, which you might recall from chapter 1 has functions in mood (the amygdala) and memory (the hippocampus).[6,7]

Research on people who have Alzheimer disease shows that music—specifically music from the era during which they grew up—not only improves mood and decreases anxiety and agitation but also increases cognitive abilities temporarily, perhaps for a few minutes or even an entire day.[8] During and after listening to familiar music, people with Alzheimer disease may be able to speak with more words, recall memories, and sing along. The documentary *Alive Inside*[9] shows the impact music can have on an individual with Alzheimer disease, including improved mood, increased awareness, clearer thinking, and reduced confusion that often occurs during the late day or early evening, which is known as *sundowning*.

STIMULATING SMELL

Aromatherapy

Aromatherapy is a relatively safe, all-natural use of essential oils to provide healing of the mind, body, and spirit. Essential oils can be used to effect olfactory (smell), gustatory (taste), and tactile (touch) stimulation. Although research has shown that a person's sense of smell may decrease as Alzheimer disease progresses, the nose is still an entryway for the sensory stimuli of essential oils because the nasal cavity and nerve cells in the nasal lining are the closest entry to the limbic system. This connection between the sense of smell and the limbic system accounts for the influence of essential oils on mood and memory.[10] Using essential oils can help in efforts to restore the body back to its natural balance. For example, if you're feeling sad, they may help you feel content; if you are feeling anxious, they may help you relax.[11,12]

Essential oils can be diffused in the air, placed on stoned jewelry, or applied to pulse points around the neck and wrist areas, like perfume or cologne. Diffusing breaks down the liquid into smaller particles, allowing them to pass through the blood–brain barrier. When diffusing essential oils, always use distilled or filtered water in your diffuser. We wouldn't want the "stuff" that's in our tap water getting into our brain. When applying essential oils to the skin, mix them with a carrier oil before application to ensure safe and effective use. Doing so cuts down on the likelihood of the most common side effect, skin irritation, and it drives the oil deeper into the skin, allowing for a faster and more effective reaction.

You will want to consult with your loved one's health care practitioner and be sure to mention any essential oils and other supplements that you may be using or want to use. Also, be sure to use a reputable product! The manufacturer should be backed by the Aromatic Plant Research Center (APRC),[13] which researches, analyzes, and tests every essential oil to ensure its purity. This information is then available for the medical and university communities and for those individuals who use essential oils regularly. Essential oils backed by the APRC have their ingredients tested and listed publicly, so you can look up exactly what is in each bottle before using it. This ensures that what you're using is the real thing.

Essential oils can work more quickly than medication taken by mouth.[11,12] When inhaled, "the absorption of essential oils by the nose is as fast as an intravenous injection [of medica-

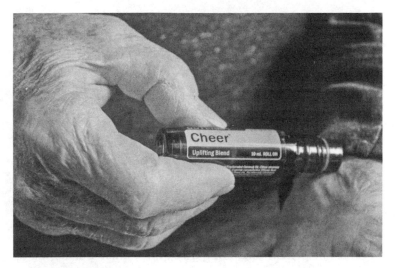

Example of an essential oil

tion]," said Gerhard Buchbauer, a professor of pharmaceutical chemistry at the University of Vienna in Austria, who has researched and documented about the chemical compounds used in aromatherapy.[25] Within 20 seconds of inhaling, an essential oil will start to work. With skin application, it takes up to 15 minutes for essential oils to reach the bloodstream, which is faster than most medications taken by mouth that have to go through the digestive system. Whether through the skin or inhalation, essential oils start to work within 2 minutes and up to 30 minutes.

Many clinical trials support the effectiveness of essential oils, including lavender and cedar for reducing anxiety and peppermint for mental stimulation.[14–16] Essential oils may also be used as part of efforts to stimulate the appetite, reduce anxiety, help with sleep, increase energy, improve attention and concentration, and much more. A published review from 2019 provides an excellent summary of studies supporting the therapeutic use of essential oils in people with Alzheimer disease specifically.[12]

It's important to keep in mind that any substance with a fragrance, including essential oils, may cause an allergic reaction in individuals with sensitivities. Use caution and test a small amount of the oil when introducing it.

STIMULATING TOUCH

Tactile stimulation occurs when we touch or are touched by an object or person, including any time we use our hands to do things. As is true for all our senses, touch stimulates neuroplasticity in the brain. In his article "What Is Brain Plasticity and Why Is It So Important?,"[17] Duncan Banks, a lecturer in biomedicine at the Open University, describes neuroplasticity as "the ability of the brain to modify its connections or re-wire itself. Without this ability . . . [it] would be unable to develop from infancy through to adulthood or recover from brain injury." In *The Dementia Concept*,[5] Josh Freitas describes plasticity as an ability to "detour around an injured part of the brain to find new ways to perform lost skills" and notes that "with the right approaches to care, people with dementia can improve neuroplasticity. Doing so can improve their cognitive abilities and slow the progression of their condition." In other words, tactile stimulation allows for greater attention and concentration in the moment.

A positive side effect of tactile stimulation is that it creates a grounding effect that helps reduce confusion and fear and lowers anxiety. Such grounding can be provided with any small exercise object, like a stress ball, hand exerciser, or fidget device. These objects provide tactile stimulation, assist with manual dexterity, increase physical activity, and improve mood.[18] Do remember that as your loved one progresses through the disease, smaller objects will become a challenge because they may try to put them in their mouth, looking for oral gratification but not knowing they can be a choking hazard, similar to the behavior of infants. Therefore, use larger tactile objects at the end of the moderate and beginning of the late stages of Alzheimer disease. Other activities that involve any form of tactile stimulation can be beneficial, like planting and gardening, knitting, sewing, arts and crafts, and even cooking or baking. All in all, tactile stimulation increases attention and concentration and lowers anxiety and fear. How great is that?

Don't Forget Taste—The Multisensory Joy of Cooking Together

Cooking or baking with your loved one is a wonderful way to meaningfully connect. Making food is an activity that uses all of our senses—touch, sight, hearing, smell, and taste. Talking about recipes and favorite dishes uses auditory senses and language skills to stimulate memories that are usually positive. Organizing ingredients and planning meals encourage the use of whatever executive functions (planning/organizing) remain, allowing for cognitive stimulation. Preparing and putting ingredients into a bowl or pot to mix engage touch. Observing how ingredients change as they are put together engages vision. The smells of cooking can stimulate sensory memories (the nose is the quickest entry to the limbic system!), which are further reinforced by the delicious taste of what you made together.

Think about how much young children enjoy the process of making things with their parents or grandparents— your loved one with Alzheimer disease can have the same sensory learning and enjoyment when they are allowed to be your kitchen helper.

If you do cook together, stay safe by ensuring there are supports for the person with Alzheimer disease and that they are protected from burners, hot spills, and sharp objects. Even if your loved one is further progressed in their disease, they can benefit from having something to hold on to, such as a wooden spoon or measuring cup, that provides the benefits of tactile stimulation discussed in this chapter.

STIMULATING MULTIPLE SENSES

Physical Activities

Physical activity has many benefits, including tactile and visual stimulation as well as improvement in overall health. If the person with dementia is listening to motivating music while exercising, then auditory stimulation comes into play. And if the individual is exercising outside, then perhaps they are smelling the outdoors and taking in a good amount of oxygen, which is great for the brain. Studies show that any level of physical activity is better for brain health than no activity[19–21] and may increase the size of the hippocampus.[22]

Pets and Therapy Animals

The unconditional love of a pet may offer a wonderful connection to someone who may not always be able to fully communicate. Pets also provide tactile, visual, and auditory stimulation, improving mood and increasing physical activity. Furry friends also assist as conversation starters. "Even people with Alzheimer's recognize a dog, and they see that the dog is someone new in their environment. I think they see it as someone with whom they can interact without any worry," says Mara M. Baun, DNSc, at the University of Texas Health Sciences Center at the Houston School of Nursing.[23]

If it is not possible or appropriate to get a real pet, try a realistic stuffed or animatronic puppy or kitten. When introducing a stuffed or animatronic animal, it is important to let the person you care for lead the way. You can approach them by saying,

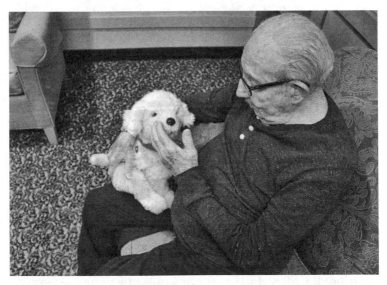

Example of a stuffed animal used as part of therapy

"What do you think about this?" The answer will likely let you know if they see it as real or not. Some individuals may know it isn't real and still enjoy it very much. At some point, however, those with dementia may think they are real and enjoy them as if they are their own pets. This makes sense according to the theory of retrogenesis; we all know small children who name their stuffed animals and enjoy them as friends.

Doll Therapy

Children light up the world of people with dementia. Depending on the activity they are doing, such as reading or playing a game, the interaction could stimulate all senses. As the disease progresses, doll therapy may prove helpful. In doll therapy, a person with dementia receives a lifelike 5- to 8-pound infant doll or mannequin to care for and nurture. Most often, the doll brings joy, unconditional love, and purpose while also providing visual, tactile, and possible auditory stimulation. A person with Alzheimer disease may care for a doll as though it is a real baby, providing the person with important daily tasks. Doll therapy may also prompt positive past memories, from when they were parents, and help them feel that they are contributing in a meaningful way.[24]

The dolls don't need to be lifelike in every way, such as wetting themselves or crying, to provide a nurturing experience for someone with dementia. Dolls with closed mouths are preferable, because your loved one won't feed them as often. Also, try to offer dolls with eyes that open and close, as this may signal to your loved one when the baby is awake or sleeping. Additionally, offer dolls that are similar to your loved one's ethnicity.

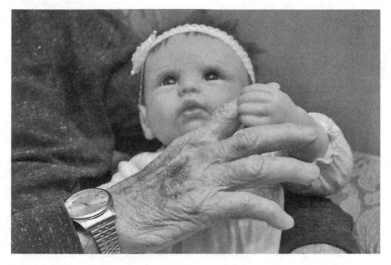

Example of a doll used as part of therapy

To add to the experience, you can accessorize—have on hand doll clothes, bottles, blankets, diapers, and so on. Your loved one will enjoy the doll more by using these tactile objects with their baby. Caring for a doll provides both tactile and cognitive stimulation, such as when your loved one is organizing the clothes by color, type, or size. A doll can provide hours of activity and can be used morning, noon, and night. The tactile and cognitive stimulation offered by lifelike dolls and pets helps to increase attention and concentration and decrease anxiety and fear.

PUTTING IT INTO PRACTICE

In retrogenesis, individuals living with dementia—just like children—can become overstimulated. It is important to limit sensory-stimulating activities and interventions to what each

41

individual can handle, which will change with time. In my experience, it is most successful to stimulate four to five senses at one time for someone early in their disease process, two to three senses in the middle stage, and one to two senses in the late stage. The best approach is to rotate senses being stimulated, so that every sense is stimulated throughout the day, maybe just not all at once. For example, if your loved one likes to cook, you might have them smell spices and talk about what dishes they might make with those spices; this is olfactory and auditory stimulation. Then, during your next interaction together at a different time, you can use those spices in a mixing exercise by putting the ingredients together, a form of tactile stimulation. Like any muscle, our brains get stronger with exercise; therefore we want to make sure we exercise all parts of it—just as we do with our bodies.

SUMMARY

The key is to interact and communicate with intention and meaning to influence your loved one's emotions in a positive way by using affirmative stimuli at an appropriate tolerance level for them. In this way, the Dementia Connection Model creates connection with purpose, love, support, and happiness. In turn, it is more likely that you, the caregiver, feel confident and happy. There is your win-win! In chapter 4, I start to share specific ways that you can use these methods for some of the challenges that many people with Alzheimer disease and their caregivers face. The goal is to fill your toolbox with as many interventions as possible!

Communication Challenges

COMMUNICATION AND RETROGENESIS

Good communication—verbal and nonverbal—is the base of all interactions with a person who has Alzheimer disease. Unfortunately, communication becomes progressively more challenging for both the cared-for individual and their caregivers. Care providers need to overcommunicate and be very good listeners. The first pillar of the Dementia Connection Model—retrogenesis—reminds us to think about how we learned to communicate and reverse it for those with Alzheimer disease. When we are born, we can communicate our need for something only by crying. As we grow, we start to use body language and facial expressions to also communicate what we need. Young parents may wish their baby could just say what they need instead of crying or acting out. A caregiver of someone with Alzheimer disease may feel the same way. The reality may be that the person you care for simply is not able to tell you what they need. Just like young parents, people providing care for those with Alzheimer disease need to observe and listen carefully to communicate well.

Communication challenges come in many forms. An individual living with dementia may have difficulty hearing high-pitched words or anything at low volume. People with Alzheimer disease—again, similar to young children—may become easily overstimulated by loud noises or by hearing several sounds at once. The vision problems that are common in Alzheimer disease can also affect communication. These difficulties include not being able to see as far or as wide, decreased depth perception, and not remembering where things are without looking. Dim light can worsen these problems. Bright or flashing lights can be overstimulating. Eventually, seeing too many colors can pose an issue for people with Alzheimer disease.

Beverly Wanders while Betty Goes Window Shopping

Beverly was walking down the hallway at the residential facility where she lived. Noticing she was near an exit and wanting to ensure her safety, a nursing assistant called to her, "Beverly, where are you going?" Beverly didn't answer. The nursing assistant asked again, "Beverly, where are you going?" but Beverly still didn't respond. Walking quickly, the nursing assistant caught up to and passed Beverly. She turned around and approached Beverly from the front, catching her eye. Suddenly, she remembered that Beverly didn't respond to that name anymore—she was using *Betty* now, the name she had been called as a girl. Now in front of her and in full view, the nursing assistant asked again, "Betty, where are you going?" Beverly said, "Just doing some window shopping, but I'm tired so I think I'll go back to my apartment now."

If a person with Alzheimer disease has dental problems or mouth pain, it can be difficult to form words. As shared in chapter 1, language is lost progressively over time. People with Alzheimer disease eventually cannot remember nouns—what people or objects are called. Later, the meaning behind what things do or who people are is also lost. Again, reversing how language is learned, people with Alzheimer disease will first speak in shorter sentences and then use only one to two words. As language is lost, body language and facial expression may remain longer but will eventually be lost toward the end of life. Then, crying out may be the only form of communication possible. Take a moment to think about where in this reversal your loved one is. That will guide you in the tools to use.

When someone is unable to use words to communicate, they may pay attention to and use more hand gestures. They may push or bat a hand away, walk or wheel away, or move objects to try to express something. They may also close and keep their mouth tightly shut or yell to communicate. Some other outwardly directed, or *overt*, behaviors include wandering off, collecting objects, repeating sounds or movements, avoiding others, and acting in an agitated or even aggressive manner. It is important for caregivers to recognize these behaviors as new forms of communication.

Next, I'll share some helpful communication tips. Recall from chapter 3 that the intention of using the Dementia Connection Model is to keep retrogression in mind and promote positive feelings in your loved one as much as possible by using affirmative sensory stimulation. Positive sensory stimulation promotes habilitation—learning through practice—at the appropriate level for your loved one's current thinking abilities. If they are happy, you are happy. Win-win!

TIPS FOR NONVERBAL COMMUNICATION

1. Use happy facial expressions, calm body language, and steady eye contact, keeping your arms at your sides or relaxed in your lap and a smile on your face. Remember, your mood is contagious. If you see that your loved one is possibly sad, first react with an empathetic facial expression to show them you understand how they feel, then attempt to cheer them up once they've seen that you understand.

2. Approach your loved one from the front. People with Alzheimer disease often have difficulty with peripheral vision and are better able to see things in front of them. By avoiding startling them from the back or sides, you can help reduce any fearfulness that may exist in the moment.

3. Use slow, steady movements. This will increase the perception of calm.

4. Use touch when it is welcomed, such as a gentle rub on the upper part of the arm or back. Avoid suddenly grabbing hands or feet, because it can be perceived as controlling or dominating and increase fear, anxiety, and agitation.

5. Demonstrate your requests with gestures. As you ask the cared-for person to do something, imitate doing it with your hands, show a picture, or use a related object. This engages habilitation—learning by mimicking and doing.

6. Praise nonverbally with nods, smiles, or a rub on the back. Everyone likes to feel praised, and a simple facial expression or hand gesture can give that. Praise encourages more positive behaviors—another win-win!

If something is just not working, walk away and try again later. It's ok to take a break so that you and the person you care for can regain control of your emotions. Just keep in mind that you will be able to try again later.

TIPS FOR VERBAL COMMUNICATION

1. Keep it simple. Use short, exact, positive phrases.

2. Speak slowly, because it gives the one you care for time to process the information you are sharing.

3. Use a warm, genuine, and adult tone of voice; don't speak too loudly or too softly. Individuals with Alzheimer disease, including those with hearing difficulties, hear a monotone and midrange volume better than a high-pitched, loud voice, which may be perceived as anger, frustration, or condescension. A warm and even-toned voice offers respect and promotes a sense of calm.

4. Use familiar words that are appropriate to the current cognitive abilities of the cared-for person. Remember, your loved one is going through the reverse of learning language, going from complex sentences to words to just crying or yelling. Eventually, the language we learned in grammar school will be their vocabulary. In middle to late stages of dementia, if you ask, "Are you in pain?" you may get an inaccurate or no response. But asking, "Do you hurt anywhere?" may elicit a different answer. If you get no for an answer and something just doesn't seem quite right, try patiently using different words to ask the same thing.

5. Give instructions for only one step at a time, and allow the cared-for person time to process and accomplish each step. For example, instead of saying, "Please put on your shoes and

coat," simplify your request by saying, "Please put on your shoes." Then, when the shoes are on, give praise and say, "Please put on your coat." Giving step-by-step instructions, one at a time, will result in better understanding by your loved one, and it will leave both of you feeling more confident.

6. Say what you are going to do before you do it. This gives the cared-for person time to prepare for what is coming and reduces fear and anxiety. One of the skill sets housed in the front lobe as part of our executive functioning skills is our ability to anticipate what comes next. As Alzheimer disease progresses, this ability becomes compromised, as discussed in chapter 1. Therefore telling your loved one what you plan to do before you do it leaves them with an assurance that the next step is safe, rather than feeling scared of the unknown.

7. Give sensory cues, perhaps by speaking about what you are doing together or by asking your loved one to help with the task. For example, when preparing a shower, ask, "Can you hold the shampoo bottle for me?" Having them hold something while conversating or completing a task will increase their compliance, because tactile stimulation increases attention and concentration and provides a calming effect. In this example, you are able to get them clean, and they are attentive, calm, and accomplished—win-win!

8. Cue frequently—at least every 15 minutes. Giving frequent sensory cues helps your loved one stay in the moment and remember what you are doing without having to rely on the short-term memory that they are losing. Try giving cues in different frequencies—every 10 minutes or every 5 minutes—to see what works for your cared-for person. When the frequency is right, confusion decreases and overtly negative behaviors are less likely.

9. Ask only one question at a time, allowing up to 90 seconds to pass before asking the next question. Just as with tasks, pauses between questions allow time for processing and succeeding with each individual question and avoids the anxiety of feeling rushed.

10. Use different forms of a person's name until you get a response. As in the story at the beginning of this chapter, people often revert to using names and nicknames from earlier in their lives.

11. Ask open-ended questions, especially in the early to middle stages of Alzheimer disease. Open-ended questions (compared to closed, yes/no questions) create opportunities to practice language, using the second pillar of the Dementia Connection Model. Later in the disease, either/or and yes/no questions may be more appropriate.

12. Give verbal praise—everyone likes to be praised. The more your loved one feels praise and validation right after doing something, the more likely the praised behavior will be repeated—that is habilitation. Repetition leads to success for that win-win!

13. Validate feelings. Let your loved one know you heard what they said. Acknowledging their words and thoughts fosters security and decreases anxiety.

14. Don't talk about the person you care for when they are in the room. Include your loved one in your conversations. Like anyone else, a person with Alzheimer disease knows when they are not included, which is likely to cause hurt feelings of being ignored or disrespected.

OTHER COMMUNICATION TIPS

1. Keep remembering to have fun. Asking a person to remember something during tasks or care can be perceived as challenging and may trigger overt behaviors. Try reserving questions about memories for fun activities, playing "Name That Tune," looking at family pictures, or chatting about old times, for example. Leave the questions intended to evaluate their cognitive level to the experts.

2. Accept the cared-for person's reality. Sadly, many people with Alzheimer disease forget life events, even when someone in the family has passed away. Although losing these memories can be painful, trying to force a person to remember doesn't make anyone feel better. Instead of reminding someone that the person they are talking about is no longer alive, you can say positively, "Tell me about a special thing [trip, date, dinner] you did together." Then the two of you can simply reminisce and talk about something you both enjoy. I'll be discussing this further later in the book.

3. Keep the environment calm. The environment can affect an individual with dementia much more easily than others. What may not seem bright or loud to you can be overstimulating to your loved one. If you notice that they are feeling discomfort or are acting out, consider whether the room is too bright, too loud, too hot, too cold, has floors that are too shiny, or has an odor. Rooms that feel crowded or overhearing conversations or conflicts can also be overwhelming for a person with Alzheimer disease. Retrogression leads people with dementia to prefer a calm environment, just like young children do.

4. Be alert for any medical issues that might be causing discomfort and may be complicated for your loved one to commu-

nicate. Hearing, vision, or dental problems; infections such as colds, flu, or urinary tract infections; and any kind of pain are likely to worsen any current problems or create new ones. Try to keep up with medical appointments as best you can to prevent any new medical concerns from developing.

5. It can be difficult for a person with Alzheimer disease to communicate that physical needs are not met in the moment. In retrogenesis, a person with Alzheimer disease may cry, call out, or use other overt behaviors in the same way that a young child does when they are hungry, tired, in pain, or need to use the restroom. You may observe that they display one kind of behavior when hungry but a different one when they are tired. All in all, you may not be told exactly what they need, but different kinds of behaviors will let you know something is wrong. Scheduling activities around meeting physical needs can be a big help; for example, taking a bathroom break every two hours and eating meals at regular times. Schedules are imperative for success, just like we try to use with young ones. Keep in mind the first of the three R's discussed in chapter 2: routine.

6. Similar to physical needs, when emotional needs are not met, overt behaviors may be triggered. Feelings of loneliness, boredom, frustration, anger, fear, or sadness will come out eventually, and you will want to pay attention to what triggers these feelings. For example, some people want to be left alone when they are sad. This could be noticed as a person lying in bed longer than usual or not wanting to leave the bedroom. Picking up on these behaviors allows you to be sensitive and give a person space or try to cheer them up with positive stimuli, using the Dementia Connection Model.

PUTTING IT INTO ACTION

In conclusion, when your loved one seems agitated, unhappy, or is displaying new or worsening moods or behaviors than usual, they may be trying to communicate something verbally or nonverbally, possibly that something is wrong. Consider everything listed above and reduce or eliminate as many triggers as you can. Going through a checklist of physical or emotional needs is a simple way to think of possible solutions to improve the situation. When you address problems and try to solve them, remember the theory of retrogenesis and communicate at a level appropriate for your loved one's ability. Use habilitation—skills-based learning—with positive sensory stimulation for success. Those three R's will come in handy— routine (consistently), remind (use sensory cues), reward (win-win!).

Let's start to build your caregiver toolbox and put these techniques into action. Use the following worksheet to write down problems or triggers you have identified that either influence or increase negative moods or behaviors—this is your loved one's new way of communicating. In the second column, write down the strategies that you plan to use to address the problem. After each attempt, put a checkmark next to the technique if it worked or an X if it did not. Try each technique at least three times. Next, switch up your technique and try a new strategy. Not every technique is going to work or work all the time. The key is to keep trying and develop as many options for success as you can—fill that toolbox. In the far right column, note which techniques you will use moving forward.

Communication/Language Challenge	Strategy Used	1st Attempt	2nd Attempt	3rd Attempt	Outcome
Seems to have difficulty understanding me when I ask if she wants something to drink	Showed her a cup and asked her	✓	✓	✓	Will continue
	Asked her at eye level, in front of her	✓	✗	✓	Will continue

Note: A checkmark means the intervention was successful; an X indicates that it was not.

Challenge	Strategy Used	1st Attempt	2nd Attempt	3rd Attempt	Outcome

Eating, Feeding, and Nutrition Challenges

EATING AND RETROGENESIS

With any activity, the theory of retrogenesis applies to people with Alzheimer disease. Think about how children learn an activity, and then reverse it for our loved ones with Alzheimer disease. Eating is no different. Babies suck and take in all nutrition in liquid form. As they grow and their strength increases and abilities develop, they hold their own bottle, sit up, and eventually eat pureed foods—first with their fingers or with someone feeding them and then on their own with a spoon. We help children learn to eat by giving them utensils that are brightly colored, easy to see, and interesting to look at. The handles are thicker than normal forks and spoons, and the material is softer than a typical adult utensil, too. Plates have dividers and larger lips for easier pushing and spooning food and better

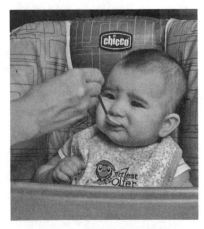

Infant eating with adult assistance

grasp. Everything is catered to meet the needs and limitations of a growing and developing child.

A person with Alzheimer disease may first have difficulty picking up and using regular dining equipment. This could be because of arthritis, carpal tunnel syndrome, or gradual loss of coordinated hand movement. Additionally, with atrophy of the frontal lobe of the brain, where problem-solving and anticipation skills reside, they are going to start to struggle with the feeding process. People living with Alzheimer disease will also have difficulty drinking from a cup without a lid. Spills may occur because of small tremors, poor grasp, or diminished hand-eye coordination or eyesight. It may be hard to gather food onto standard utensils with regular plates.

In the moderate to late stages of Alzheimer disease, your loved one may no longer remember what utensils are called and eventually lose the meaning behind what they do. Remember the verbal cueing discussed in chapter 4. Gentle reminders to use the fork can help the person you care for maintain the skill of using utensils for longer. Eventually, though, it will become too difficult for the person living with Alzheimer disease to use utensils at all. Gradually, the individual will use their fingers to put food in their mouth and then will stop eating independently and need to be fed by caregivers. Late in the disease, even swallowing becomes a challenge.

Mary's Mom Doesn't Have to Eat Like the Baby

Remember Mary's mother Joyce from chapter 2? Joyce was struggling with using regular utensils, and her daughter was frustrated that she would hold a spoon in one hand while picking up the food and eating with her other hand.

Mary noticed that her mother was eating the same way her granddaughter did. But I could tell that Joyce still had the ability to feed herself because she could hold a spoon in one hand. I recommended that we give Mary's mom utensils that were easier to use and have one of the specialty therapists work with Joyce to relearn her eating skills. With this approach, Joyce was able to maintain eating with utensils for quite a while longer. This intervention kept Joyce at a higher level of independence for as long as possible. Eventually, Joyce transitioned to eating more bite-sized foods, which were easier for her to eat yet also allowed her to feed herself.

Along with difficulty eating, the environment, meal, and timing may also be challenging for a person with Alzheimer disease. Your loved one may be overwhelmed or potentially even under-stimulated by the environment. Bright or dark lights, loud sounds, room or food temperature changes, chaos, negative or minimal interactions, and so on can all distract or deter the cared-for person to not want to eat. Even the amount of food on a plate can be overwhelming. Because problem solving and decision making have become more difficult, a person with Alzheimer disease may not be sure how to start the meal or may become easily distracted from eating. Initially, serving meals in courses is ideal, as it cuts down the amount of food to choose from to get started. As the disease progresses, however, the timing of the meal may need to go back to being served all at once, or you may need to stay right next to your loved one during meals to show them the next food item. Doing this will help keep the eating process going and minimize the chances that they get up or think the meal is over after one serving.

Let's talk about some tools you can use with your loved one to help with eating, feeding, and nutrition. With every skill, remember the Dementia Connection Model and try to promote positive feelings with affirmative sensory stimulation for habilitation—learning through practice. And the more consistently you do it (routine), using sensory cues (remind), the more independent your loved one will remain and the more accomplished you'll feel (reward)!

TIPS FOR EATING, FEEDING, AND NUTRITION

In 2016, I conducted a focus group with people with varying dementias, implementing the techniques listed below together in a dining program. We looked at meal consumption, weight, and use of supplements as markers for this three-month trial, in which we trained the staff and prepared the study. By the end of the trial, 46% of residents increased their consumption of food. In addition, 54% of residents either gained or maintained weight. At first, 18% of residents were using supplements because they weren't consuming enough food. By the end of the three-month period, though, only 5% of the population were using supplements.

The Eating Environment

1. Make sure the area where your loved one eats is comfortable. Take note of the temperature, sound level, lighting, and mood of the environment. Make adjustments as necessary for optimal comfort. People with Alzheimer disease have difficulty concentrating, so keep the environment from being too overwhelming

or distracting. Lighting is especially important because many people with Alzheimer disease have vision issues that can make it difficult to see the food on the plate or as it moves toward their mouth. Just take care not to make the room too bright, which would make them uncomfortable, or too dim, which may put them asleep. Just as important is to ensure the temperature in the room is comfortable. Uncomfortable temperature may encourage your loved one to want to leave the room or become agitated. Just think about if you are too hot or too cold—not fun.

2. Make sure your loved one is comfortable, checking to see whether they need to use the bathroom before eating or have any pain or discomfort that needs to be addressed, like stomach issues or body aches. Bodily discomforts can easily distract someone from eating.

3. Address your own comfort and mood, too! Remember, your approach and mood are contagious, and a positive attitude creates an easygoing, calm, and even fun atmosphere. As discussed in chapter 1, your loved one can still experience an array of emotions, even if it is difficult to express them. Eating is a main activity, repeated several times a day—we all want it to be pleasurable.

4. Play music your loved one enjoys. This will provide auditory stimulation and help create a serene environment. The type of music can vary, depending on the situation or time of day. Try upbeat music with words in the morning to ignite verbal skills. People with Alzheimer disease can often sing along or hum music they know, increasing and encouraging language. Consider upbeat but less familiar music for lunch, which may help them focus more on conversation. At dinner, consider chimes or a single tone to help your loved one relax in preparation for nighttime.[1]

5. Sit directly in front of your loved one. Diminished eyesight, depth perception, and peripheral vision make it difficult for a person with Alzheimer disease to see people and objects that are not directly in front of them. If you need to be next to them to assist or feed them (see "Feeding" later in this chapter), sit on the side of the hand they use most often. Sitting on this dominant side creates a comfortable and natural experience, because our dominant side is where we have more control over things.[1]

6. Have a complete setup for each meal. A completely set table and the routine that goes with it offer visual stimulation that reinforces the skills-based knowledge and procedural memory of eating. This habilitation can be further reinforced by having your loved one set or help set the table, if able. Setting the table provides visual and tactile stimulation and provides a continued sense of purpose.

Mealtime Routines

1. Try to have meals at consistent times, and establish a set routine leading up to and following meals. For example, before every meal, use the bathroom, wash hands, set the table, and sit down. Because people with Alzheimer disease gradually lose planning and organizing abilities (the executive function skills discussed in chapter 1), a mealtime routine helps with task starting and sequencing. After consistently following a routine for four to six weeks, your loved one will likely participate freely because they will have learned it—this is the first of the three R's.

2. Have the same easy-to-hold and bright utensils at every meal to avoid confusion and sustain interest. When it is unclear

what utensils mean or do, a person of any age or ability will be unlikely to use them. If you are unaccustomed to chopsticks, for example, you're likely to opt instead for the fork next to your plate. Familiarity and routine foster continued independence and control to help a person feel confident and dignified. If your loved one reaches a point where they can't use utensils but can and want to eat with their hands, offer finger foods.

3. Use the same dishes at every meal, preferably bold-colored ones to catch attention, draw interest to the food, and help make it more visible. As discussed in chapter 3, colors make a difference.[2,3] Red can increase food consumption by 25%, and yellow sustains attention. Much like brightly colored dishes and utensils appeal to children, such dining ware may help people who are experiencing retrogression.

4. Make things easier by serving and eating a little bit at a time, as mentioned above. People with Alzheimer disease can be easily overwhelmed, even by having three or four foods on a plate instead of one or two. After success with one food, you can give praise and then serve more or another food. Keep in mind though, as the disease progresses, you may need to go back to serving the meal all at once or to providing one course after another to avoid confusion.

Taste and Smell

1. Use sweet flavors such as applesauce or ketchup for dipping or dabbing onto food. Taste buds change over time, and people with Alzheimer disease may prefer flavors from their early childhood. When we were young, most of us avoided bitter, savory, or strong flavors—preferring sweeter foods like applesauce over broccoli, for example. Therefore, to get the

cared-for person to eat their broccoli, dabble some applesauce, or even ketchup, on it.

2. Food that has a strong smell can be distracting or overwhelming. Consider using scents that stimulate the appetite and improve mood, such as citrus essential oils diffused in the air. If your loved one seems agitated at mealtime, a lavender-scented essential oil can be calming.[4,5] Even if your loved one has a diminished sense of smell, taking in the scent through the nasal passageway still provides a natural and effective benefit to the body.

Feeding

Most people with Alzheimer disease will eventually need to be fed or, at the very least, given physical assistance as they feed themselves.

1. Sit in front of or on the side of whichever hand is used most often (the dominant hand). People with Alzheimer disease lose peripheral vision over time and can have difficulty seeing people and objects that are not right in front of or right next to them.

2. Use the hand-under-hand technique[6] of cupping your hand under your loved one's dominant hand while they and you hold the utensil together. This technique provides support and guidance for their movements. Additionally, the act of holding both the utensil and your hand prompts tactile stimulation, which increases attention and concentration and lowers anxiety and fear.

3. Another option could be to allow the person you are feeding to hold your wrist while you use the utensil. Grasp is one of the first reflexes a person experiences. In retrogenesis, grasp

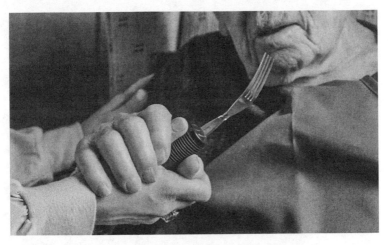

Example of feeding using the hand-under-hand technique

is likely to be the last reflex to be lost, or it may not be lost at all. Letting someone hold your wrist and feel your movements engages skills-based learning and procedural memory. Again, this increases attention and concentration and lowers anxiety and fear through tactile stimulation.

Other Helpful Tips

1. Remove any wrappers before serving food to your loved one. In the late stages of Alzheimer disease, this is especially important because even condiment wrappers may be confused as food items. The hand dexterity for removing wrappers also diminishes as the disease progresses.

2. Use verbal cueing. As discussed in chapter 4, good communication creates a strong base for all other activities. As you assist with meals, feeding, and nutrition, periodically tell your loved one what you are doing or, when possible, have a conversation related to the meal at hand. Such cues will continuously

remind the person that they are eating, minimizing confusion about what they should be doing or where they should be.

3. Give positive reinforcement and praise. I've said this before and will say it again. Everyone enjoys compliments. When you praise the behavior, it is more likely to be repeated, in turn continuing to make caregiving easier. Win-win!

4. Changed eating patterns should be discussed with your loved one's doctors. A decrease or increase in appetite can have causes that you will want to investigate first (for example, side effects from medications, infections, pain, or dental issues).

5. Be as consistent as possible. If the environment, routine, music, and essential oil scents are a consistent, daily occurrence, after about four to six weeks, your cared-for person will learn it is time to eat when those interventions are used.[7] A routine will help them become more aware and participate in what's happening, increasing the likelihood that they eat, and you will have reassurance that they are getting the nutrition they need. Win-win! This approach constitutes the three R's discussed in chapter 2—routine, remind, reward. It can be used in other areas of care that we will be discussing, like bathing and sleeping.

PUTTING IT INTO ACTION

Let's put these techniques into action. On the following worksheet, in the left column, write down the challenges you and your loved one face during meals and snacks. This may take some time, so observe and pay attention to the little nuances around the room. Trust me, it will be all worth it once you figure out their triggers! Next, write down the strategies that you plan to use for each challenge. Then, after each attempt, add a checkmark if it worked or an X if it did not. Try each technique at least three times, and be sure to switch up your technique and try something else. Not every technique is going to work for every individual or all the time. The key is to keep trying. I'm going to help you slowly build your toolbox of interventions. Look at all those checkmarks and determine which techniques were a win-win; those are the techniques you will use moving forward.

Eating Challenge	Strategy Used	1st Attempt	2nd Attempt	3rd Attempt	Outcome
Dad is not eating very much	Served one portion at a time	✓	X	X	Will not continue
	Switched to red plates	✓	✓	✓	Will continue
	Diffused citrus essential oil in the air	X	✓	✓	Will continue

Note: A checkmark means the intervention was successful; an X indicates that it was not.

Challenge	Strategy Used	1st Attempt	2nd Attempt	3rd Attempt	Outcome

Sleeping Challenges

SLEEP AND RETROGENESIS

Sleep needs and patterns change as Alzheimer disease progresses, once again in a reversal of childhood development. The individual will start to sleep more during the day than at night, taking one and then two naps a day. In the late stage of the disease, a person with Alzheimer disease will sleep most of the day.

Lack of good-quality sleep, however, can cause irritability and restlessness, especially in the mornings if sleep did not occur the night before. This also causes a worsening sleep pattern by making a person so tired the next day they have more daytime sleep, only to be more awake that night than the previous night. Poor sleep also worsens pain and makes all activities of life more difficult,[1] and the more a person gets out of bed at night, the more opportunities they have to fall or hurt themselves. The bottom line is that we all need sleep, regardless of age or condition, but a good night's sleep is even more important for people with Alzheimer disease, much like it is for infants.

As a caregiver, I recommend that you first focus on what your loved one's current sleep pattern is like. In the sleep patterns I have observed in people with early-stage Alzheimer disease, they usually sleep through the night unless there are problems unrelated to Alzheimer disease affecting sleep. People with early-stage Alzheimer disease may not take naps or take only one nap each day, and they sleep typically six to eight hours a night. In mid-stage Alzheimer disease, people usually take one or two naps during the day and sleep four to six hours each night. Nighttime sleep tends to decrease as the disease progresses. In the later stages of Alzheimer disease, they will take two or more naps throughout the day, and their nighttime sleep may be as little as two to four hours per night. Take a moment to think about where your loved one is in this pattern. If you're not sure, consider keeping a sleep diary.

Betty's Bedtime Routine

Every night, Betty preferred to be tucked in with a kiss on the forehead and her companion pet tucked in by her left side. The caregiver routinely said, "Good night, Betty. We will see you in the morning." Betty then slept soundly throughout the night. We found, however, that when a caregiver did not follow this routine, Betty got up several times a night, leaving her irritable and restless the next day.

If your loved one's sleep pattern does not match the stage that they are currently experiencing, then it is beneficial to discuss the issue with their doctors. Sleep can be disturbed for several reasons unrelated to the disease itself. It's best to get this checked out.

One thing to be mindful of is that individuals with dementia can get bored easily during the day, causing them to fall asleep unnecessarily. Boredom may cause a person to do unproductive things such as wandering aimlessly, collecting objects, or even napping. These behaviors are hallmarks of under-stimulation. Sleeping too much during the day when it's not appropriate for a person's stage of disease can cause unnecessary difficulty sleeping at night, and even more concerning is that under-stimulation can cause a decline in their cognitive processes. Compare the sleep pattern of the person you care for to what is described above and consider whether it is typical for the stage of the disease they are experiencing.

As care providers, we want our loved ones to have a good-quality sleep to elicit a positive mood. By using the Dementia Connection Model, you can help ensure they get a good night's sleep through the use of affirmative, positive stimuli. Remember, it's best to use the three R's—routine, remind, reward.

TIPS FOR GOOD SLEEP

The Sleep Environment

The National Sleep Foundation recommends that all individuals have a consistent and comfortable sleep environment that is used primarily or exclusively for sleep whenever possible.[2]

1. Keep the bedroom cool, between 60 and 67 degrees Fahrenheit, for optimal sleep.

2. Turn off bright lights and avoid using backlit devices such as cell phones, televisions, or tablets, which are known to disrupt sleep. Consider hanging blackout curtains to ensure the room stays dark.

3. A nightlight can be used if your loved one is not fond of complete darkness or tends to get up in the middle of the night

and needs to see. A motion-sensing nightlight is ideal, providing safety and comfort when your loved one is awake enough to move about, but turning off so that sleep is not disrupted once a person does get back in bed.

4. A comfort item to hold on to or lie next to can provide the tactile stimulation and security discussed in chapter 3. This can be a companion pet, doll, blanket, or special pillow.

5. Using calming music or a white-noise machine can provide calm auditory stimulation. White noise can also be provided by a fan or humidifier set to a comfortable sound level.

6. Lavender essential oil can help promote a deep sleep with olfactory stimulation.[3] If used, it should be diffused throughout the night and not just for a few hours, so that sleep is not disrupted. If the cared-for person does not like the smell of lavender, try another scented essential oil. Roman chamomile, sandalwood, and frankincense are good alternatives. In my experience, women tend to like flowery scents, and men tend to prefer woodsy scents.

The Bedtime Routine

The National Sleep Foundation also recommends that all individuals, not just children and people with dementia (the first pillar of the Dementia Connection Model), follow a sleep routine, also known as sleep hygiene.[2] For individuals with dementia, a sleep routine activates the second pillar, habilitation, which is learning through practice. If you follow the same routine for four to six weeks (the first R) using sensory cues (the second R), the one you care for will learn to associate it with sleep and benefit from feelings of comfort, safety, predictability, and calmness, which constitute the third pillar and the third R.

1. Going to bed around the same time every night and waking around the same time each morning are proven to help people get enough sleep.[1]

2. Start 30 minutes before bedtime by limiting light exposure and stimulation. Avoid conversations that may be upsetting. Begin the process of calming down for sleep knowing that everyone takes time to relax.

3. Ensure your loved one's bodily needs have been met before going to bed. You will especially want to make sure that they have used the bathroom before lying down.

4. Teeth brushing and face washing provide sensory stimulation (taste, touch, and smell) that will help engage habilitation and be part of a healthy bedtime routine.

5. Provide a comfort object and tuck your loved one in if that is their preference (tactile stimulation), promoting attention and concentration and lowering anxiety and fear.

6. Use verbal cueing (discussed in chapter 4) as a mode of auditory stimulation that promotes routine learning. Statements such as "Let's get ready for bed" and "See you in the morning," repeated the same way every night, as in Betty's story at the beginning of this chapter, can be helpful.

Other Sleep Tips

1. Natural light exposure during the day has been shown to promote healthy sleep and to offer other health benefits.[4,5] There is also evidence that light therapy may have positive effects on brain metabolism and cognition in people with Alzheimer disease.[6]

2. Exercise during the day. Even 10 minutes of aerobic exercise per day has been shown to help people get a good night's

sleep.[2] I also recommend starting the day with more high-intensity activities to use up energy during the day and promote sound sleep at night. This could mean physical activity in the morning after breakfast, such as taking a walk or playing some fun games like trivia in the midmorning. Try to expend energy both mentally and physically in the morning, with less stimulating activities in the afternoon. This allows the body to naturally come down throughout the day, getting the brain and body ready for sleep at night. Don't have your loved one exercise just before bed. Exercise can act like a stimulant and make it harder to fall asleep.

3. Avoid caffeinated beverages, sugary items, and other stimulants, including nicotine, at dinnertime and afterward. All of these are known to disrupt sleep. Drinking alcohol too close to bedtime should also be avoided; even though it may help a person relax initially, alcohol can disrupt sleep later in the night when the body begins metabolizing the alcohol.[2]

4. Address any pain that is keeping a person awake as proactively as possible. Work with your loved one's doctors to ensure that healthy pain management strategies are in place, and stick to them.

5. Remember that your own mood makes a difference. People experiencing retrogenesis learn by mimicking, so if you are calm and peaceful at bedtime, the person you care for is more likely to be as well. If you are having a bad evening, ask someone else to help. If there isn't anyone who can help in the moment, take some slow and steady deep breaths or perhaps consider using lavender essential oil to calm yourself before starting the bedtime routine.

6. If your loved one gets up during the night, calmly redirect

them back to their room. Use verbal cues and reminders that it is still nighttime and that you'll see them in the morning.

7. If you notice changes in sleep patterns, consult your loved one's doctors. Changes in sleep patterns, like changes in eating patterns discussed in chapter 5, may not have anything to do with Alzheimer disease. Sleep changes can be the result of taking new medications, a sign of depression, or a symptom of an infection, other illness, or undiagnosed or unmanaged pain.

8. Continue the bedtime routine even when clocks and seasons change, remembering that these changes can disrupt anyone's sleep but that it shouldn't last for more than a couple of days or weeks.

PUTTING IT INTO ACTION

Are you ready to put these techniques into action? On the following worksheet, in the left column, write down the challenges that your loved one currently has with sleeping, such as having difficulty getting to sleep or staying asleep. In the next column, write down the strategies that you plan to try. After you have tried a strategy, put a checkmark next to it if it worked or an X if it did not, and be sure to try each strategy at least three times. Then, switch it up and try a different technique. Don't rely on only one strategy. You want to fill your toolbox with lots of great interventions. Remember, not every technique is going to work for every individual or all the time. The key here is to keep trying and then determine which techniques you plan to use moving forward.

Sleeping Challenge	Strategy Used	1st Attempt	2nd Attempt	3rd Attempt	Outcome
Mom can't fall asleep	Companion pet	✓	X	X	Will not continue
	Diffused lavender essential oil	✓	✓	✓	Will continue
	Bedtime routine	X	✓	✓	Will continue

Note: A checkmark means the intervention was successful; an X indicates that it was not.

Challenge	Strategy Used	1st Attempt	2nd Attempt	3rd Attempt	Outcome

Toileting Challenges

TOILETING AND RETROGENESIS

As explained by the theory of retrogenesis, a person with Alzheimer's will have difficulty remembering to use the toilet and start to have accidents. People with Alzheimer disease will slowly lose the cognitive signal related to the feeling of having to go to the bathroom. As the disease progresses, incontinence will occur. Wearing incontinence briefs and needing assistance with toileting will become necessary at some point.

Other environmental factors can be related to incontinence concerns. Sometimes, being assisted by family members from a younger generation or caregivers of the opposite sex can make an individual feel uncomfortable or embarrassed. Such embarrassment may lead to being secretive about using the toilet, which can then lead to accidents. Uncertainty or confusion about when and where to use the toilet can lengthen the time it takes to reach a toilet, which can also lead to accidents.

No one wants to feel embarrassment or shame over simple bodily functions. For the person you care for, it is important to promote positive feelings around toileting as much as possible. Routinely use the Dementia Connection Model to influence emotions in a positive way through the use of affirmative stimuli.

TOILETING TIPS

The Toileting Environment

1. The bathroom should have a comfortable temperature—not too cold or too hot.

2. The lighting should be bright enough for a person to see well, but not so bright as to overwhelm. Consider using a motion-sensitive light in the bathroom for use during the night.

3. Provide a high-contrast colored toilet seat (recall from chapter 3 that bright-colored objects are easier to see for people with Alzheimer disease).

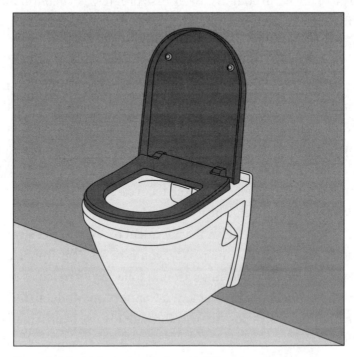

Example of a high-contrast colored toilet seat

4. Make use of visual cues, such as placing a sign on the bathroom door that looks like a toilet to remind your loved one where the bathroom is. The most effective signage is printed in clear typefaces and large (22 to 24 point) sans serif fonts with bold accent colors.[1,2]

5. People with Alzheimer disease may also respond well to signs placed next to the bed or a favorite chair that remind them to use the bathroom. In the later stages of the disease, this will be a less effective tool if the individual no longer has the ability to read or has poor eyesight when reading.

6. Leave the bathroom door open when not in use so that your loved one can see the toilet—a visual reminder of what the room is for and where to go to the bathroom—and ensure that there is easy access to the bathroom. At some point, you may need to remove the door to the bathroom to provide a wider angle to see the toilet.

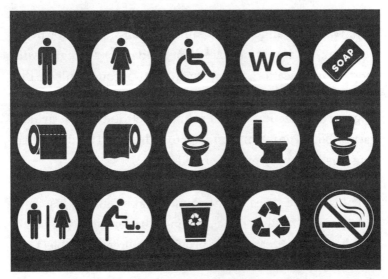

Examples of visual cues to consider for bathrooms

7. Consider installing grab bars by the toilet to help your loved sit down and stand up, minimizing their risk of falling while using the bathroom.

Toileting Routine

1. A toileting schedule is one of the best tools you can make to help your loved one avoid accidents. Ask and assist them to use the bathroom at least every two hours. A proactive toileting schedule helps to avoid the negative feelings and discomfort of accidents.

2. Ensure the person you care for is drinking plenty of fluids, preferably water, so that they are successful with regularly scheduled bathroom breaks. Men need about 15 cups (3.7 liters) of water a day; women need about 11 cups (2.7 liters).[3] Staying hydrated also helps prevent urinary tract infections, which can lead to a series of medical, cognitive, emotional, and behavioral challenges.

3. Watch for any signs of pain, and consult a doctor if you see them. Because your cared-for individual struggles with good communication, it may be difficult to communicate that they feel pain, like when urinating or defecating, which can be a sign of an infection or other illness. Left untreated, urinary tract or bowel problems can lead to kidney and bladder infections, making everything more difficult.

4. Use positive reinforcement and praise immediately after your loved one takes a bathroom break. You can also promote positive feelings by scheduling a preferred activity right after bathroom breaks or by providing a preferred object immediately afterward. This gives auditory, tactile, and visual stimulation as well as reassurance that they have done a good

thing. You are simply reinforcing what they should be doing—something that people with Alzheimer disease often struggle to do.

Other Toileting Tips

A person with Alzheimer disease may forget they just went to the bathroom and ask to use it again. To avoid this situation, the experience of going to the bathroom has to be meaningful and connected to sensory information and procedural memory, two of the three pillars of the Dementia Connection Model.

1. You can note the sound of the toilet flushing. I know that sounds funny, but it really works! The sound and your verbal cue give good auditory stimulation. You can simply say, "The sound of the toilet is really loud [soft], isn't it?"

2. For tactile stimulation, you can ask the person you care for to hold on to the toilet paper or wipes for you, if you assist with wiping.

3. Diffusing peppermint or rosemary essential oil provides olfactory stimulation. These scents may be helpful in efforts to improve focus and concentration.[4–6]

4. Do not scold your loved one for having accidents or react negatively when accidents occur. Your loved one did not intend to have an accident and certainly didn't want it to happen. Scolding or reacting harshly creates a negative tone around toileting that sets you both up for more negativity. Remember the win-win, and be as reassuring as you can.

5. Continue having a routine of using the bathroom even if your cared-for individual is using incontinence briefs. Keeping this routine can help maintain a level of independence and dignity.

6. Consult your loved one's doctor as needed, especially if incontinence occurs when taking a new medication, as this can be a side effect. Some illnesses and infections can also cause incontinence.

7. Refer to any incontinence products used as an "incontinence brief," or simply "brief," rather than "diaper." Referring to these products as diapers can be shaming and embarrassing for the cared-for person.

PUTTING IT INTO ACTION

Let's put these techniques into action with a worksheet. As in earlier chapters, write down in the left column any challenges that your loved one currently has with toileting (if they don't have these problems yet, you can always come back to this at a later time or use the approaches proactively). Then note the strategies you plan to use. After you have tried a technique, put a checkmark next to it if it worked or an X if it did not. Try each technique at least three times, and switch up your techniques to see what else works. The key, as always, is to keep trying.

Toileting Challenge	Strategy Used	1st Attempt	2nd Attempt	3rd Attempt	Outcome
Accidents	Toileting schedule	✓	✓	✓	Will continue
	Increased fluid consumption	✓	✗	✓	Will continue

Note: A checkmark means the intervention was successful; an X indicates that it was not.

Challenge	Strategy Used	1st Attempt	2nd Attempt	3rd Attempt	Outcome

Bathing Challenges

BATHING AND RETROGENESIS

As Alzheimer disease progresses, individuals lose the skills needed to take care of themselves. With our understanding of retrogenesis, we know that bathing skills for people with Alzheimer disease are lost in reverse order of how children learn to bathe themselves. First, everything is done by the parents as they wash an infant in a tub (or in a basin in the sink with a sponge). As children become able to sit and play in the tub, they may hold the soap and then gradually be encouraged to wash themselves. Later in childhood, they learn to shampoo their own hair and take showers. By adolescence, bathing is done independently, although reminders may be needed.

Reversing that for a person with Alzheimer disease, we understand that, at first, they will need reminders to shower, then assistance with showering, followed by a preference for baths with assistance, and eventually sponge baths in bed. Keep in mind, if the goal is to get someone clean, how it is done doesn't matter. Your loved one may have difficulties with problem solving or understanding why bathing is necessary. Other bathing challenges for your loved one with Alzheimer disease may include fatigue, forgetfulness about what bathing items are called or what they are used for, and trouble communicating. All of these factors can make your loved one more likely to become overwhelmed, overstimulated, or refuse care in the moment. Other factors that can occur for any adult who needs care include feeling fear, anxiety, embarrassment, or a loss of control.

Dolores's Day

For years, Dolores followed a morning routine where she woke up, put on her bathrobe and "house shoes," and went to the bathroom before starting any other part of her day. When her daughter made the decision to move Dolores into a residential facility, we sat with both of them to get to know Dolores better. We replicated her daily routine to ease the transition and make her feel right at home.

Dolores also liked to brush her teeth when bathing. When brushing her teeth, Dolores only needed assistance with taking the cap off the toothpaste and putting the toothpaste on her toothbrush. We used the hand-under-hand technique discussed in chapter 5, which helped her feel as though she was doing it all by herself. We sometimes even brushed our teeth with Dolores, providing visual stimulation so she could still see how to get to the back of her mouth and clean behind her teeth.

Dolores was still able to shower independently— mostly. Her "window of opportunity," as we called it, was up to seven minutes. By six minutes, we would use verbal cueing with words that would help her remember what she was doing. During her shower, we would provide tactile and auditory stimulation by asking, "Dolores, can you hold the shampoo bottle for me? That would be so helpful!" With this cueing, she would not forget what she was doing and remained calm. Also, Dolores would often sing with us in the shower, with lead vocals by her favorite caregiver—"I'm singin' in the rain, just singin' in the rain"—which helped increase cooperation and fun. Win-win!

After Dolores was almost ready for the day, she always had to put on her favorite lipstick and the necklace her late husband gave her when they first started dating. When she would put it on, we would say, "Dolores, your necklace is so beautiful!" Dolores would reply and with a wink of her left eye, "He's a keeper," referring to her husband.

With this positive reinforcement through auditory, tactile, and visual cues, Dolores would know her bathing routine was complete, and move on to the next part of her day.

With some simple techniques, many of these obstacles can be minimized for your loved one living with dementia. Using the Dementia Connection Model consistently, you can influence emotions to be positive using affirmative stimuli during the bathing process. The three R's will be handy during bathing—routine, remind, reward.

BATHING TIPS

Below are some tips guaranteed to help experience a win-win in relation to bathing. If you use these tips in succession, you are utilizing the three R's of routine, remind, reward. By using a consistent bathing schedule and sensory cues to influence positive emotions, your loved one benefits and so do you. Win-win!

The Bathing Environment

1. Ensure that the temperature in the bathing area is comfortable.

2. Check that the lighting is bright enough that your cared-for person can see easily and safely, especially if they are doing things independently, but not so bright that they are overwhelmed or unable to relax while bathing.

3. Use items or products that are contrasting in color and not too dark, which will help with visual stimulation. Colored and contrasting towels and bathmats are useful. Avoid white; white items tend to be seen as a blur by people with Alzheimer disease.

4. Consider the scents of bathing products and remember that these will offer olfactory stimulation. For morning showers, diffuse essential oils that are invigorating, like peppermint or a favorite citrus scent; for evening baths, lavender can promote relaxation. Perfumed products may cause skin irritation, so using essential oils is preferable. As always, be alert to any allergic reactions to essential oils.

5. Play calming music or use a white-noise machine for positive auditory stimulation while bathing. Songs from the era a person grew up in that are meaningful to the individual tend to work best. You can also sing or play a song that your cared-for individual likes at every bathing experience, as we did with "Singin' in the Rain" for Dolores. By repeating the same song with consistency, routine skills-based learning—habilitation—will be engaged, making future bath times more likely to be positive.

6. Make sure all products and items needed are within arm's reach so that you do not leave your cared-for individual alone

in the bathing area, creating an unsafe gap in care and potentially causing fear and anxiety or, worse, slips and falls.

The Bathing Routine

1. As with all caregiving activities, your mood is infectious. Maintain a calm and positive attitude, with a smile on your face for positive visual stimulation. You want your loved one to mimic this attitude and demeanor. Win-win!

2. Remember to approach your loved one from the front or from their dominant side. As discussed in previous chapters, the vision and concentration problems of Alzheimer disease make it difficult for people to see what is not directly in front of them. Approaching from the front avoids startling a person and diminishes fear and anxiety. When you can't approach from the front, being on your loved one's dominant side will feel more familiar and in control.

3. Check that the needs of your cared-for person have been met as much as possible before starting. Any pain, thirst, or need to use the toilet should be addressed first. If a person did not sleep well the night before, consider delaying bathing.

4. Try the hand-under-hand technique described in chapter 5, but only if needed, where you cup your hand under theirs, encouraging and guiding their hand to pick up the soap or shampoo. This technique provides tactile stimulation that is calming and seems noncontrolling and more natural, which can help increase cognition and decrease anxiety.

5. Allow your cared-for individual to do any part of bathing they can independently. Continuing to practice a skill for as long as possible helps the person keep that skill for as long as possible, but keep in mind that eventually even these skills will

be lost. Also, remember that if you do more for a person than is needed, you may create excess disability.

Other Bathing Tips

1. Use verbal cueing throughout bathing, saying what you are going to do before you do it. The auditory cue provides warning of what is coming next and helps minimize any fear. Be careful to provide only one instruction at a time (as discussed in chapter 4) so that the cared-for individual has time to process and succeed before moving to the next step. Cueing is needed at least every 15 minutes, and it is helpful to learn the timing, or "window of opportunity" as we called it for Dolores, for each individual and use that as your cueing interval.

2. Giving a person something to hold during bathing increases attention and concentration and decreases anxiety.

3. Use a back-to-front technique for rinsing the head and hair. Start pouring water at the base of the back of the neck, moving over the head and to the front of the forehead. This helps a person know to close their eyes before the water reaches their face, making rinsing the head and hair less bothersome or overwhelming. Do not pour water directly on the face.

4. Provide positive reinforcement during bathing, such as saying, "You look great!" or "Great job!" If you find that a particular phrase gets a positive response, you can use it over and over to encourage habilitation—sensory-stimulated procedural learning—and increase the likelihood of more positive bathing experiences.

PUTTING IT INTO ACTION

Now that you've learned several techniques, let's put them to the test. On the following worksheet, in the left column, write down the challenges that your loved one currently has with bathing. Next, write down the strategies that you plan to use. After you have tried the technique, put a checkmark next to it if it worked or an X if it did not, and be sure to try each technique at least three times. Finally, try a new technique (for example, taking a bath instead of a shower or having them hold the shampoo bottle). Not every technique is going to work with everyone or work all the time. The key is to keep trying. After trying several different techniques, determine which ones you will use moving forward and note those for your toolbox.

Bathing Challenge	Strategy Used	1st Attempt	2nd Attempt	3rd Attempt	Outcome
Doesn't like water poured on her face	Pour water from back of head to front	✓	✓	✓	Will continue
	Give her the loofah to hold on to	✓	✓	✓	Will continue

Note: A checkmark means the intervention was successful; an X indicates that it was not.

Challenge	Strategy Used	1st Attempt	2nd Attempt	3rd Attempt	Outcome

Pain and Pain Management

As discussed in chapter 4, it can be difficult for individuals with Alzheimer disease to express their senses and emotions. Pain is highly subjective, with each individual having their own threshold of tolerance. More than half of people with any kind of dementia, including Alzheimer disease, regularly experience pain.[1] There is evidence suggesting that people with Alzheimer disease have a higher subjective (expressed) pain threshold and a lower biological threshold.[2,3] That is, they experience relatively more pain and express relatively less pain. This disconnect makes addressing any pain that is expressed nonverbally—and especially verbally—of utmost importance.

Again, retrogenesis applies: children first cry and react physically to pain before learning to express it verbally, ask for help, or independently manage pain. Conversely, people with Alzheimer disease first lose the ability to manage their own pain (problem solving), then the ability to ask for help (communication), and eventually can only react to pain. Pain reactions are often aggressive, such as yelling out repeatedly, hitting, or biting. It is important to consider whether pain is the cause of any of these behaviors and address pain before assuming it's anxiety (more on that in chapters 10 and 11). Often, instead of considering pain as the cause, the individual is treated from a psychiatric standpoint, such as being prescribed antipsychotic or antianxiety medications, to treat the behavioral issues.

Untreated pain makes aggressive behaviors worse and can result in using increasingly higher doses of psychiatric medications that do not address the underlying pain at all. These medications also have many potential side effects.

To help your loved one with any pain they may be experiencing, observe their behavior closely, always consider the possible need for pain management before changing other aspects of care, and use the Dementia Connection Model to influence emotions positively with affirmative stimuli. Good pain management is a win-win, making the cared-for person both more comfortable and easier to care for.

George's Leg Hurts, but He Says He's Not in Pain

George was receiving physical therapy services in one of our communities. During a session, the physical therapist noticed George wincing and moaning a bit. George also was rubbing his right upper thigh, over and over again. He stopped following directions and wouldn't engage in the rest of the therapy session. The therapist first thought that George was displaying odd and resistive behaviors but quickly realized that he seemed to be in pain. The therapist asked, "George, are you in pain?" George shook his head no. His response perplexed the therapist because he looked and acted as if he was in pain. She rephrased the question and pointied to his leg, "George, does your leg hurt?" George quickly replied, "Yes!"

TIPS FOR PAIN MANAGEMENT

Pain Assessment and Treatment

1. Observing any nonverbal signals of pain is even more important than asking if your loved one is in pain or hurts somewhere. Moaning, grunting, sighing, or crying out are all ways of expressing pain. People may also rub or grab body parts that are painful or withdraw from a touch. Movements may be slower, and posture may be rigid. People in pain are more likely to cry, get frustrated or angry, seem irritable, or have changes in sleep or appetite.

2. The memory of previous pains may still be very real for a person with Alzheimer disease. They may also experience confusion about areas of current pain. For example, if your cared-for person fell and broke a hip five years ago or had a knee strain last year, those body parts may still ache today. Talking about past pain may be easier than talking about a new pain. Keep previous incidences of pain in mind, and be sensitive to those areas while looking out for possible new pain.

3. When asking about pain, use simple language and ask things in more than one way, just as George's physical therapist did. You can ask, "Do you hurt?" or "Does ___ hurt?"

4. Consult your cared-for individual's health care providers for proper treatment of pain and any conditions causing pain. Give any medications exactly as they are prescribed. Your loved one's doctors should avoid prescribing opioids, because these drugs have side effects on cognition and more. They are also highly addictive. A daily dose of acetaminophen may be all it takes to address your loved one's pain. Ask their doctor before starting any new medication or pain management regimen.

5. Before trying a new drug, talk to the doctor about treatments that do not use medication.[3] These nondrug treatments include physical therapy, exercise that is appropriate to an individual's abilities, applying ice or heat to the area (depending on preference), easy stretching, light massage, or diaphragmatic breathing paired with progressive muscle relaxation. All of these treatments provide tactile stimulation, and exercise in particular may benefit cognition.[4-6] Over-the-counter pain relievers, such as acetaminophen or ibuprofen, can be helpful after exercise to prevent pain and may make it easier to continue an exercise program.

6. I have found the use of essential oils—especially turmeric, frankincense, rosemary, or peppermint—beneficial as part of a plan to help loosen muscles and alleviate pain. Essential oils should be mixed with a carrier oil of choice, such as coconut or jojoba oil, and then applied topically directly to the site of pain for tactile stimulation. If your loved one has a headache, then the essential oils could be smelled for olfactory stimulation—which is effective in some.

Tips to Prevent Worsening of Pain

1. Good sleep quality is important for anyone experiencing pain, because poor sleep worsens pain, and pain disrupts sleep. The American Academy of Sleep Medicine recommends seven to eight hours of sleep per twenty-four-hour period for healthy adults. People with Alzheimer disease may need more sleep than that and often need to nap during the day. See chapter 6 for information on helping the individual you care for get enough sleep.

2. Pain, anxiety, and depression often occur together. Being overly anxious or depressed can cause aches and pains in the body, and pain can cause an individual to feel anxious or depressed. Therefore any feel-good activities can distract your loved one from their pain issues. Using techniques discussed in previous chapters that use affirmative stimuli to promote positive feelings can be helpful. See chapter 3 for an overview.

3. Avoid any rigorous movements immediately upon waking in the morning. Your loved one may be achy from the night's sleep, or they might just need a little time to adjust to getting up. Avoid prompting any rough movements of the body to avoid furthering pain or negative feelings.

4. Another option is palliative care, a service that is usually provided by a home health or home care agency. The goal of palliative care is to provide symptom relief, improving quality of life for both the individual with Alzheimer disease and their family.

PUTTING IT INTO ACTION

Let's put these techniques into action! On the following worksheet, in the left-hand column, write down your loved one's possible areas of pain. Next to that, note the strategies that you plan to use to treat their pain (ice or heat, massage, essential oils, etc.). After each attempt, put a checkmark next to the technique if it worked or an X if it did not. Try each technique at least three times, and switch up your techniques to see what else is effective, keeping in mind that nothing will work for every person every time. Keep trying new techniques and decide which ones you will keep in your toolbox.

Pain Challenge	Strategy Used	1st Attempt	2nd Attempt	3rd Attempt	Outcome
Pain in legs	Light massage	✓	✓	✓	Will continue
	Icing areas of pain	✓	✓	✓	Will continue

Note: A checkmark means the intervention was successful; an X indicates that it was not.

Challenge	Strategy Used	1st Attempt	2nd Attempt	3rd Attempt	Outcome

Depression, Hallucinations, and Delusions

DEPRESSION

Depression is common for individuals living with dementia. Although the exact causes of depression in Alzheimer disease are unknown, changes in brain chemistry clearly play a role. Brain chemistry changes may be triggered internally by aging, genetics, or another disease, such as Alzheimer's. External factors such as experiencing the death of a family member or friend, life changes, or other traumas and stressors may also trigger changes to brain chemistry, which can lead to depression.

Understanding these external factors and the role that brain chemistry plays, it is not that surprising that up to 40% of people with Alzheimer disease have depression. We know their brains are changing (retrogression) because of the degeneration and atrophy that are part of Alzheimer disease (see chapter 1). People with Alzheimer disease also experience changes in their lives as their abilities change. Symptoms of depression can include sadness, tearfulness, loss of pleasure in activities that used to be enjoyable, feelings of guilt, difficulty concentrating, weight loss or gain, sleep disturbances, and thoughts of death.

If the person you care for appears to be experiencing depression, they should have a visit with their physician. Your loved one's health care provider can carefully assess whether depression or something else is going on and refer you to other specialists if needed. It is important to be clear and straightforward with the physician about what you are observing in the person you care for so that proper treatment can be started.

Kathleen's Necklaces

Our resident Kathleen really enjoyed wearing her costume necklaces every day, and we knew it was just the thing she needed to keep her depressive and anxious symptoms at bay. Kathleen had a history of experiencing depression on and off throughout her life. Her children told us that they recalled from their childhood that their mom never really felt sure of herself and often put herself down. Kathleen initially exhibited similar symptoms when in our care, often asking if she looked ok, commenting on her weight, or repeatedly inquiring about what she should be doing or where she should be going, often followed by weeping. When we introduced the pearl necklaces, knowing she loved to dress up, her eyes lit up. Once she put them on, her demeanor completely changed. She seemed like a new, confident, vibrant woman. We also observed that Kathleen played with the necklaces in between her fingertips. The tactile stimulation seemed to quiet the anxiety she was experiencing. She appeared calm and content when wearing her necklaces. When Kathleen did not wear them, we all noticed an increase in her sadness, worry, and self-doubt.

TIPS FOR HELPING WITH DEPRESSION

You can use the Dementia Connection Model to support a loved one with Alzheimer disease who is also depressed. As presented throughout this book, using positive and affirming sensory stimulation can help improve mood for both of you. Here are some strategies that may be particularly useful.

1. Encourage or assist your loved one to engage in routine physical activity. Endorphins, our natural mood elevator, are released in the brain during exercise. Additionally, physical activity can provide tactile stimulation, increasing attention and concentration and decreasing any anxieties or fear. Any exercise—such as going outside for a walk—will stimulate the senses (sight, smell, and hearing). Research shows that regular physical activity can improve cognition in people with Alzheimer disease and is protective against depression.[1-3]

2. As discussed in chapter 3 and incorporated into the tips in many other chapters, playing music that your loved one enjoys can reduce anxiety and improve mood.[4-6] Singing along, especially to music from the era during which your loved one grew up, may be especially beneficial.[7]

3. Art therapy has been shown to have benefits for both Alzheimer disease and depression.[7] This cathartic activity has been shown to relieve symptoms of depression and anxiety. Coloring is an easy way to incorporate artwork into day-to-day activities and provides tactile and visual stimulation.[8] Therefore, it can improve mood while also increasing attention and concentration and lowering anxiety. Artwork also creates opportunities for shared experiences with nonverbal communication; the person can express themselves artistically when they can no longer find the words to do so.

4. Going back to Kathleen's story at the start of this chapter, something as simple as verbal praise (auditory stimulation), such as saying, "You look beautiful in your necklaces," can go a long way toward improving someone's mood.

5. Other uplifting approaches include inviting pets to come around or having someone or something to care for, like a doll, both of which were discussed in chapter 3.[9,10]

6. Aromatherapy provides olfactory stimulation; citrus scents specifically can help to improve mood and therefore may be useful in treating symptoms of depression.[11] These scents can be diffused in the air (lasting up to four hours after the diffusing stops), or you can apply drops to diffuser jewelry (lasting up to eight hours). Additionally, you can apply essential oils to pulse points around the neck (lasting for four hours), or even apply a couple drops to all-natural felt furniture pads ("personal diffuser dots"), which you can stick under your loved one's lapel or on the inside of their collar by the neckline (lasting up to eight hours).

7. If your loved one is in the earlier stages of their disease, they may benefit from talking to a counselor or psychologist about how they are feeling. This can give them an outlet to vent and process what they are going through while providing cognitive stimulation through the therapeutic process. Occupational therapy may be another option. Enhancing their motor skills may help your loved one feel more confident in their abilities, boosting their self-esteem and decreasing feelings of depression.

8. If the cared-for person is spiritual, leaning on their faith may be what they need to help them through what they are feeling. They may find that talking to a chaplain or priest is therapeutic.

9. Getting your loved one back to doing their favorite activities can be beneficial. Gardening, cooking, or baking can help improve mood through the positive sensory stimulation that such activities provide.

HALLUCINATIONS AND DELUSIONS

Individuals with moderate to advanced Alzheimer disease might see or hear things that aren't there (hallucinations) or believe things that aren't true (delusions). This can be part of the course of Alzheimer disease (described in chapter 1), but observing either of these behaviors in your loved one should trigger a visit to the physician the first time it happens. Your loved one's health care provider needs to know about delusions or hallucinations. There could be other causes that need treatment, and paying attention to how delusions and hallucinations change over time is an important part of understanding how your loved one is doing. Not all individuals who have Alzheimer disease have these experiences, but many do.

Often, some delusions and hallucinations begin as a person with Alzheimer disease relives a moment from the past as if it was happening right now. For example, a person might believe they have to go to work or that their children are small, not realizing that the grown adult standing before them is one of those children. Or they may mention having spoken to their mother, who you know passed away 10 years ago. Remember, they are experiencing retrogression, and their reality may be what happened 10 years ago or even 50 years ago. They may also get stuck in this time frame for quite a while—all pretty normal occurrences as the disease progresses.

What Does It Mean to Live One's Truth?

Peter often provides care for his friend John. One day when he arrived at John's apartment to take over from another caregiver, John was dressed in a suit and tie and looking for his briefcase. Instead of telling John that he hadn't worked as a lawyer for many years, Peter said, "We're taking the day off together today to go to the park. Then we're going to grab a bite at your favorite diner." John smiled and said, "That sounds great!" John changed into comfortable leisure clothing, and he and Peter went for a walk in the park. During the walk, Peter asked John to tell him which of his many cases he had found most challenging as a lawyer. They had a healthy breakfast at John's favorite diner and walked home, both feeling calm and happy.

TIPS FOR DEALING WITH HALLUCINATIONS AND DELUSIONS

1. Live their truth. As we touched on in chapter 4, and as Peter did for John in our story, if the one you care for is having delusions, it is best to stay in the moment and "live their truth." This doesn't mean accepting their delusion as your reality; it means you don't contradict them or say that what they are experiencing isn't true. Correcting or arguing with a person with Alzheimer disease will only create conflict and negativity, especially because to them the delusion or hallucination is simply quite real. After all, at some point in the past, it likely happened. The

goal is to navigate the situation so that the end result is your loved one feeling happy and you feeling at ease. Win-win!

2. When your loved one is experiencing a hallucination or delusion, redirect the conversation so that whatever your loved one is remembering or thinking about is discussed in a positive way. For example, if your loved one is talking about a parent who has passed away as though they were alive, you can ask them to share stories about what their parent did for them when they were a child. This creates an opportunity for verbal communication and connection without challenging your loved one's reality.

3. Practice makes perfect. Your loved one's false sensory perceptions or belief systems will usually remain the same, so you will have time to try multiple different responses. Use responses that work for you and them; these will typically be your go-to's when they are expressing these experiences.

4. If these symptoms seem to make your loved one feel sad, then utilize the strategies listed above. If your loved one is feeling frustrated or angry, however, see chapter 12, which discusses feelings of aggression.

You need to take care of yourself if you want to take care of your loved one effectively (more on this in chapter 13). It is hard to see the person you know and love slipping away slowly, increasingly referencing a past that you weren't present for. They will forget, in succession, their great grandchildren, grandchildren, children, and then husband/wife or partner last. Remember that your loved one does not have control over this retrogression and likely would prefer to remember all they can—including you. Check with local hospitals to see if any offer free support groups for family members of those with dementia. You can also look up support services or references on my website, NeuroEssence, at neuroessence.org or on the Alzheimer's Association website at alz.org. Don't be afraid to seek psychotherapy or counseling for yourself if you need it.

PUTTING IT INTO ACTION

It's time to build that toolbox if your loved one is or has experienced depression, hallucinations, or delusions. Even if your loved one hasn't experienced these symptoms yet, it is still a good idea to plan ahead and sketch out what you would do in the event it comes on all of a sudden. On the worksheet below, in the left column, write down the challenges with depression, delusions, or hallucinations your loved one is having now. If there are none, you can skip to the next column, where you'll write down the strategies you will or think you might use. After you try a technique, put a checkmark next to it if it worked or an X if it did not, and try each technique at least three times. Don't forget to switch up your technique to see what other strategies (for example, playing music, diffusing essential oils, or introducing a companion pet) might work. You can't have too many tools in your caregiver toolbox.

Mood Challenge	Strategy Used	1st Attempt	2nd Attempt	3rd Attempt	Outcome
Depression	Companion pet	X	X	✓	Will not continue
	Artwork	✓	✓	✓	Will continue
	Diffusing a citrus scent	X	✓	✓	Will continue

Note: A checkmark means the intervention was successful; an X indicates that it was not.

Challenge	Strategy Used	1st Attempt	2nd Attempt	3rd Attempt	Outcome

Repetitive Behavior, Rummaging, and Collecting

REPETITIVE BEHAVIORS AND RETROGENESIS

Repetitive behaviors consist of verbal or physical actions that are repeated over and over, like saying phrases such as "help me, help me" or making hand gestures like clapping. Take into account the theory of retrogenesis. Children repeat themselves verbally and physically, and as dementia progresses, your loved one may do so as well. Just as in children, these repetitive behaviors and chants are often related to an underlying sense of being uncomfortable or feeling not in control (like being in pain, not having basic needs met, feeling negative emotions, or being overstimulated).[1,2] Typically, if your loved one has repetitive behaviors, those behaviors will be consistent throughout the disease process. The helpful part of this symptom is that you will get to know what that behavior is telling you and how to intervene.

Rummaging or collecting may occur for a number of reasons, including perceptions that the items are valuable or fears of forgetting where things are. This behavior is a characteristic of retrogenesis, much like toddlers collect items around the house, and parents have to find their hiding places.

Maria's Tapping and Typing

At mealtimes, Maria would repeatedly tap her fingertips on the dining room table. Others around her would stare or get frustrated, but Maria would keep tapping until a plate of food was placed in front of her. Then she would stop.

During her move-in evaluation, her daughter informed us that Maria had been a stenographer for the court system. We realized that Maria was acting as though she was at a desk and seemed to believe she was at work each time she was wheeled up to the dining room table. She tried "typing" with her fingertips whenever she was at a table or what she believed was a desk.

Maria was simply acting out of habit because of what she did for a living for so long. The act of typing seemed to satisfy a need to feel purposeful. In order to minimize Maria's confusion and the frustrations of other diners at her table, we ensured she had a plate of food waiting for her at meals, providing visual stimulation that showed her it was time to eat, not work. We also developed a "life-skill station" for her that included a desk and a typewriter for more visual, tactile, and auditory stimulation, which she used intermittently throughout her day. Maria would spend hours typing away. These interventions helped boost her self-esteem, reduced her repetitive symptoms, and seemed to make her and others happy. Win–win!

TIPS FOR REPETITIVE BEHAVIORS

Using the Dementia Connection Model, when your loved one exhibits repetitive behaviors, try to meet their basic needs first, with retrogression in mind, because often the behavior is caused by thirst, hunger, tiredness, pain, or a need to use the bathroom. Next, think about habilitation, as your loved one can still experience a wide range of emotions and will make sense of the world around them through their senses. Using positive, affirming sensory stimulation and a calming demeanor can help to minimize the repetition in the moment. This approach can have a positive effect on a number of senses, influencing your loved one's emotions and helping them to feel happy, secure, and comfortable.

1. If your loved one is asking the same question over and over, answer calmly, as if it was being asked for the first time, every time. Your loved one may mimic your calm, cool, and collected auditory and visual stimulation.

2. Avoid scolding or getting frustrated. If you need a minute to take a deep breath before responding, then do so. Remember, they are regressing to an earlier age.

3. Recall that tactile stimulation reduces anxieties, so introducing a pet, baby doll, or weighted blanket across the lap can be helpful.[3]

4. Diffusing or smelling essential oils provides olfactory stimulation for a calming effect in some people. Rosemary, lavender, and Roman chamomile may be particularly helpful for calming.[5,6]

5. Distraction with food, conversation, or activities of interest can minimize repetitive behaviors.

6. Playing soothing or mood-boosting music can also help calm repetitive behaviors. You can even play some white noise to calm the cared-for person. White noise is what we heard in our mother's womb—it becomes very soothing again for an individual with dementia.

7. If your loved one makes repetitive sounds, working with a speech therapist can help alter what the cared-for person is saying to use words that aren't so alarming or stress-provoking for you or those around them.[4] For example, the statement of "help me, help me" can be changed to "you and me"—this simple change sounds much more friendly and inviting. Remember that through these verbalizations, your loved one is trying to tell you something but cannot find all the words to tell you, similar to when an infant cries or says the same thing over and over to get their needs met. The words your loved one says aren't as important as you observing and discovering what the meaning of those words are.

8. Allow your loved one to collect items safely by purposefully putting out items that are safe and putting away items that are not. Be careful to ensure that what you put out is not small enough to be put in the mouth, as small objects are a choking hazard. Allowing the behavior to occur safely may provide needed visual and tactile stimulation. Collecting can be rewarding and even provide a sense of purpose. Some find purple items to be more likely to be hoarded, as purple is a sign of royalty, so take this into consideration if you do leave collectible items out.

PUTTING IT INTO ACTION

Repetition can easily be managed with the right tools. So, let's put these techniques into action. On the worksheet below, write down your loved one's repetitive behaviors in the left column, and next to that, list the strategies you plan to try (such as food, music, dolls). Then, after you have tried a technique, add a checkmark each time it worked and an X each time it didn't. Try each technique at least three times, and keep trying different techniques to see which ones work for you and your loved one. Nothing will work for everyone or every time, so keep trying. The silver lining with repetitive behaviors is that they tend to stick with a person, so you are likely to figure out what they mean and master managing these behaviors over time.

Behavior Challenge	Strategy Used	1st Attempt	2nd Attempt	3rd Attempt	Outcome
Says "Help me" repeatedly	Doll	X	✓	✓	Will continue
	Diffusing lavender scent	✓	✓	✓	Will continue

Note: A checkmark means the intervention was successful; an X indicates that it was not.

Challenge	Strategy Used	1st Attempt	2nd Attempt	3rd Attempt	Outcome

Sundowning, Aggression, and Wandering

SUNDOWNING AND RETROGENESIS

Sundowning, a worsening of symptoms and behaviors in the late afternoon or early evening, is common in individuals with Alzheimer disease, although not all experience sundowning. Anticipation of night without awareness of when it will come is thought to be a factor. When sundowning occurs, the individual is more confused, irritable, sometimes aggressive, and may wander more than usual. Like most people, the later it gets in the day, the more tired an individual becomes; for people with dementia, however, it is much more difficult to handle. Remembering retrogenesis as part of the Dementia Connection Model is useful—just as children are more likely to lose their self-control when they are tired, so too are people with Alzheimer disease. Typically, this happens around the same time every day for an individual.

TIPS FOR SUNDOWNING

Sundowning can be minimized and even eliminated. Being proactive with the Dementia Connection Model by using approaches about 30 minutes before sundowning usually begins can make a tremendous difference. As always, use sensory stimulation and skills-based learning (habilitation) to make the approach to sundowning a positive habit. The three R's—routine, remind, reward—must be used here in order to try to minimize or eliminate sundowning. Below, I call this the "perfect day."

1. Have a consistent waketime and bedtime to promote healthy sleep so that a person is less likely to be tired during the day. (See chapter 6 for more on sleep.)

2. Schedule exercise and other higher-intensity activities in the morning rather than the later afternoon. Starting the day with physical activity can boost mood but expend energy.

3. Getting enough light in the daytime is also critical to getting enough sleep (see chapter 6). Going outside daily for about 30 minutes, whenever weather permits, provides sensory stimulation and promotes healthy sleep. Exposure to daylight helps reset a person's circadian rhythm and its clear delineation between day and night. During the winter or times of inclement weather, using a light box of at least 10,000 LUX for 30 minutes every morning can help achieve sufficient light exposure.

4. Taking rest periods throughout the day can help minimize sundowning. As discussed in chapter 6, the number of rests or naps needed will increase as a person's Alzheimer disease progresses. Schedule rests into their day (one in the morning and/or one in the afternoon), and follow that schedule daily. As long as your loved one is engaged in between these rest periods and not sleeping too much during the day, their naps should not interfere with nighttime sleep. These rests can serve the body and brain and also provide caregivers with a break. Win-win!

5. About 30 minutes before their sundown time, use tactile stimulation as a calming technique. This may include time with a pet, snuggling a companion or baby doll, or using a weighted blanket.

6. The olfactory stimulation of essential oils can also be calming for some, especially if using rosemary or lavender.[1,2] Diffuse these oils into the air about 30 minutes prior to sundowning.

7. Try playing music at the same time you are using your tactile objects or diffusing essential oils. Music can help create a feeling of calm.

Implementing the three R's—routine, remind, reward—daily for four to six weeks using "the perfect day" method will help your loved one respond positively to your interventions. In time, they will respond automatically or within seconds to minutes each day, which may completely eliminate the sundowning effect.

AGGRESSION, WANDERING, AND RETROGENESIS

Retrogenesis tells us that even coping skills will reverse. We are all born with a biologic fight-or-flight response to stress that gives us the ability to defend ourselves (fight: aggression) or run away from (flight: wandering) danger. Even very young children have these reactions, and as they grow they learn to control them, fighting or fleeing only when something is life threatening and not each time they feel alarm or distress. That process for your loved one with Alzheimer disease is reversed, meaning that they will gradually become less able to control the urge to fight or flee; aggression and wandering may occur as a result.

Verbal and physical aggression can be triggered by feeling scared, angry, tired, or overstimulated. Not having needs met, communication difficulties, confusion, pain, or hallucinations and delusions can also trigger aggression.

Wandering may be aimless, with your loved one not knowing where they are going or why, or goal-directed, as when a person is trying to get something for themselves or trying to find something but may not know where or how. Wandering can be triggered by the need to leave a confronting, negative, or scary situation or to meet basic needs. Mimicking someone who was leaving or hallucinations and delusions may also trigger wandering. A lack of structure or routine in the day and feelings of boredom can increase confusion and cause more wandering.

TIPS FOR AGGRESSION OR WANDERING

To prevent aggression or wandering, try to determine what is triggering this behavior and reduce that trigger. It may take some time to observe and understand connections between the behavior and what happened right before or around the same time the behavior occurred. These tips can be used proactively to reduce wandering and aggressive behaviors in the moment, to deescalate aggression, or to stop wandering.

1. If your loved one becomes confused in any given moment, after a certain number of minutes, use the communication approaches of cueing with verbal, visual, and tactile cues around a minute or two before that time frame passes (see chapter 4).

2. If aggressive behavior or wandering occurs when your loved one is hungry or needs to use the bathroom, try to note (or even keep a diary for one to two weeks) how often this occurs (for example, every three hours), and then schedule meals or bathroom breaks before the aggression or wandering is likely to occur (for example, every two to two and a half hours).

3. Remember that being overstimulated (or under-stimulated or bored) can trigger confusion and fear that may lead to aggression or wandering. If the environment is too stimulating, take your loved one to a calmer, quieter, less bright area. If boredom is the issue, try to engage your loved one in a positive activity to influence a positive mood. Tactile activities are great because they increase attention and concentration and lower anxiety.

4. Your mood undoubtedly affects the mood of your loved one. If you are becoming frustrated or irritable yourself, take a break if you can. Try to do something that calms you down, such as deep-breathing exercises or saying something to yourself to boost your mood. If you have to walk away and try again later, then do it.

5. Another approach that I find successful is offering an either/or choice, which communicates respect and gives control to the individual with dementia. As the caregiver, you control the two choices offered, allowing boundaries and limits to what you will engage in, use, or have. For example: "Do you want to wear the red or green shirt today?"; "Do you want one or two creamers in your coffee?"; "I know you are upset. Do you want to talk here or over there?" Giving predetermined choices can help deescalate aggression, prevent wandering, and even eliminate these behaviors when used proactively.

6. Auditory stimulation with white noise, another soothing sound, or music can be calming (as discussed in chapter 3) to address aggression.[3-5] Instrumental music, especially music that features just one instrument, can be calming to a person with dementia. Choose music the person you care for recognizes and enjoys, which will engage them and reduce wandering. Make it meaningful, for that positive auditory stimulation ultimately connects the two of you.

7. Use tactile stimulation with pets, dolls, or weighted blankets to calm your loved one or give them a reason to sit instead of wander.[6]

8. Schedule exercise as part of a daily routine so that your loved one's need to move is met. Exercise can proactively burn off stress and anxiety. It also helps prevent depression (see chapter 10) and improves sleep (see chapter 6), lessening daytime tiredness that can lead to aggression or wandering.

9. Avoid drawn-out goodbyes, or stop saying goodbye altogether. The phrase may lead to aggression (to get you to stay) or wandering (trying to follow you) because your loved one does not want to be alone or even left with someone other than you. People with Alzheimer disease worry about being separated from their loved ones, just like small children often have fear when dropped off at school or left with a babysitter. Because of retrogression, your loved one may not have any real sense that you will return.

10. Lavender essential oil for olfactory and possibly tactile stimulation also may be used as part of a strategy to calm an individual with dementia.[1,2] Place it on pulse points, diffuse it, or put a couple of drops on stoned jewelry or a "personal diffuser dot." Additionally, if there is a certain time of day that your loved one tends to wander or become aggressive, utilize

lavender about 30 minutes to an hour before then to reduce the likelihood of either behavior. If your loved one doesn't seem to care for a certain scent, try another oil or another method.

11. Show compassion and empathy, and validate your loved one's feelings.[7] Avoid any use of force, including trying to make a person who was wandering be still. This compassion toward your loved one can help diminish the fight-or-flight response.

PUTTING IT INTO ACTION

Let's put these techniques into action. On the following worksheet, the first column is for the behaviors your loved one has (sundowning, aggression, or wandering), the second column is for the techniques you'll try, and next to that are columns for marking whether a technique worked (checkmark) or didn't (X) and whether you'll continue using it. Try each technique at least three times. As always, switch up techniques to find out what works for you and your loved one. Nothing will work for everyone all the time. Recall that when it comes to sundowning and aggression/wandering, you are trying to change behaviors related to a natural process and an innate coping skill, respectively, which may take some time and remain challenging. The key is to keep trying. Now, fill that toolbox.

Behavior Challenge	Strategy Used	1st Attempt	2nd Attempt	3rd Attempt	Outcome
Aggression	Giving limited options	X	✓	✓	Will continue
	Diffusing lavender scent	✓	✓	✓	Will continue

Note: A checkmark means the intervention was successful; an X indicates that it was not.

Challenge	Strategy Used	1st Attempt	2nd Attempt	3rd Attempt	Outcome

Intentional Care

I hope that what you've read so far has been helpful in expanding your understanding of Alzheimer disease and learning how the Dementia Connection Model can improve your caregiving. If you've been using the worksheets, you will have tried the model several times and documented what worked for you and your loved one. Some of the approaches you tried may not have been successful, but some may have helped a lot. Photocopy, take pictures on your smart phone, or remove the pages with successful strategies and put them on the fridge, a bulletin board, or some other place that you can reference easily—this will be your toolbox. Continue to use these approaches to help make win-win situations, those that influenced emotions in a positive way, making you and your loved one happier. Don't forget to come back to the workbook if your loved one develops new symptoms.

SELF-CARE AND SOLITUDE

Part of successfully connecting time and time again with your loved one using the Dementia Connection Model is to be intentional—focusing on the needs and wants of your loved one—from a place of compassion. Finding that compassion day in and day out requires some solitude and self-care. Simply put, you have to take care of yourself in order to successfully take care of your loved one. Self-care is easy to talk about but often hard for caregivers to do. I conducted a focus group in May 2019 and learned the following information about caregivers.

- 55% said they have *struggled with self-care* at some point in the past

- 45% answered they have *lost touch with their hobbies* or don't have a hobby

- 60% responded they spend so much time taking care of others that they *don't take time to care for themselves*

- 40% answered that at times they *feel guilty when caring for themselves* because they could be caring for others

Flight attendants review the safety procedures before take-off. Part of their review is to explain the function and use of oxygen masks, which will drop from overhead if the airplane loses cabin pressure. The airlines remind all of us to secure our own oxygen mask before helping others, because you won't be able to help anyone if you can't breathe yourself. The same is true in life. If you don't take care of yourself, you will eventually be unable to care for others. That is not a win-win.

TIPS FOR SELF-CARE

1. As a caregiver, you need to find outlets that help you destress in order to feel fresh and ready to connect intentionally every day, or the days that you are providing care. Think about what

you do for fun or what makes you feel relaxed. Schedule hobbies, events, and self-care appointments on your calendar so that you do not forget or get too busy to do them.

2. I recommend taking an hour a day for yourself. Now, you may be thinking, "How could I possibly find an hour a day for myself? I work or take care of mom, and I have children to pick up from school and dinner to make for my family. It just isn't possible." It is possible. There are 24 hours in a day; you choose what you do with those hours. Adjust, adjust, adjust. You can choose to wake up one hour earlier than usual or go to bed one hour later. You can choose to take that one-hour lunch break that your company gives you instead of working through it, as so many of us often do. You can choose to use the time when the person you care for is sleeping to do something for yourself.

3. If taking an hour seems like too much, try a shorter time frame, like 15 minutes. Take 15 minutes a day for yourself to do some deep-breathing exercises, which can help you focus and stay calm. Take 15 minutes to go for a brisk walk or run, which will help increase your endorphins, improving your mood and energy. Take 15 minutes to enjoy your coffee or tea in peace, perhaps outside, watching and listening to the birds to calm yourself.

4. Influence your own emotions by using affirmative stimuli. You're worth it and you need it. What scenery calms and soothes you? What sounds make you smile? Do you have a favorite scent? What music makes you want to dance? Who makes you smile as soon as you see them? Do you have a favorite food? What do you like to do with your hands? As you schedule breaks for yourself, try to find time to look, listen, smell, taste, and touch these things. Your brain responds to sensory input and learns from it, too. Don't forget to connect with yourself!

5. If a friend or family member offers assistance, accept the meals they make for you, or watch a movie you enjoy together. Take them up on their offers of help. You are not burdening them, and taking them up on their offer doesn't say anything about you, other than you are willing to fill your cup so that you can continue to fill your loved one's cup, too.

AVOIDING BURNOUT

Feeling overly stressed day in and day out can lead to burnout, which can mean different things to different people. Generally speaking, burnout is a feeling of being emotionally and physically depleted.[1] Burnout can cause a caregiver to become detached from the person(s) for whom they provide care.

Burnout can cause the caregiver to act in ways they are not proud of, like having a short fuse, yelling at their loved one, and sometimes even displaying violence. Burnout also overlaps with and can cause depression. People experiencing burnout may not care for themselves well or turn to negative coping skills, like drinking excessively or using drugs, driving recklessly, getting into fights with others, and even exhibiting suicidality.

Research suggests that finding meaning in the care you provide to someone else can prevent burnout.[2] Take time to think about the gift of time and care that you are giving your loved one. What would it mean if you were not willing and able to do that? How would it affect not just the one you care for but also the other people in your lives? What beliefs motivated you to take on the role of caregiver? Staying in touch with the answers to these questions, along with taking time for yourself, can keep burnout at bay.

PUTTING IT INTO ACTION

This journey of Alzheimer disease is not an easy one. There will continue to be good days and bad days. But let the number of bad days decrease and the good days increase. Self-care will allow you to be purposeful and intentional every time you are caring for your loved one with dementia. Use the worksheet to apply the Dementia Connection Model to yourself. Yes, I want you to log your successes too, just like you would when caring for your loved one. In the left column, write down some of the things you miss or wish were easier. Then note some sensory-focused ways you can address those issues, like using essential oils, gardening, adult coloring, listening to music, and the like. After you've tried one, add checkmarks or X's to keep track of what does and doesn't work for you. Try each technique at least three times, and keep trying different things. Then, take your planner or smart phone and schedule those self-care activities for the next 30 days. Start with one or two tools and then add another after 30 days. You deserve and need care, too, and when you have it, you will be better able to care for others— win-win!

Self-Care Challenge	Strategy Used	1st Attempt	2nd Attempt	3rd Attempt	Outcome
Guilt	Journaling	X	✓	✓	Will continue
	Diffusing citrus scent	✓	✓	✓	Will continue

Note: A checkmark means the intervention was successful; an X indicates that it was not.

Challenge	Strategy Used	1st Attempt	2nd Attempt	3rd Attempt	Outcome

Promoting Brain Health

Many people fear that they will develop dementia, especially if they are caring for a family member with Alzheimer disease. Some risk factors, such as age and genetics, we can't change. The good news is that there are actions we can take that can reduce or eliminate other risk factors for Alzheimer disease: inactivity or lack of exercise, heart disease, diabetes, social isolation, low education levels, poor sleep, excessive alcohol or drug use, smoking, and limited cognitive and sensory stimulation.[1-4]

First, I'm going to share actions *known* to reduce risk. We know these methods work not just because many studies have shown that people who did these things are less likely to develop Alzheimer disease but also because additional research—called meta-analysis—has evaluated all studies together to look at the quality and reliability of that research. Second, I will also share ways to address factors being studied as possible risks. Finally, I'll touch on the need to carefully evaluate claims that something will protect you from Alzheimer disease.

KNOWN METHODS TO REDUCE
DEMENTIA RISK

1. Keep your heart and blood vessels healthy. Your brain is only three to four pounds of your entire body weight but receives

20% of your blood flow and the oxygen it delivers. A healthy brain requires oxygen and blood flow, and a healthy heart is needed to deliver them. Strokes and mini-strokes can cause vascular dementia and also increase the risk of Alzheimer disease.[1-4] If you smoke or use tobacco products, work with your health care team to stop. Together, keeping your blood pressure, cholesterol, weight, and blood sugar at healthy levels with a nutritious diet and exercise, and medication if needed, can set you up for success.

2. Exercise regularly and maintain a healthy weight to improve your heart health and reduce the risk of heart attacks and strokes that are bad for the brain. Some studies suggest that exercise and a healthy weight reduce the risk of dementia independently of positive effects on the heart, making these actions even more important.[5-10] The second edition of the US *Department of Health's Physical Activity Guidelines for Americans* suggests that adults do a minimum of 150 minutes of moderate-intensity exercise or 75 minutes of aerobic activity per week, including muscle strengthening activities for all major muscle groups. Adults over age 55 should include balance training in their exercise regimen.[11] All people should consult with their health care team before starting a new exercise program, especially if they are not exercising regularly already.

3. Several studies have shown that a heart-healthy diet—such as the Mediterranean diet—may reduce dementia risk.[12-15] Whether this is because of benefits to the heart or to both the brain and heart is not yet clear, but since a healthy heart promotes a healthy brain, following one of these diets may be a good idea.

A Heart- and Brain-Healthy Diet

High in fruits and vegetables

High in nuts and legumes

High in whole grains

Low-fat dairy products

Low salt

Skinless poultry and fish

Nontropical vegetable oils

Limited saturated fats and no trans-fats

Limited sweets and no sweetened beverages

Limited or no red meat (leanest cuts available)

6 oz. of red wine daily

Plenty of water

4. Diabetes is a known risk factor for dementia, which may be because of damage to blood vessels from diabetes or because of the importance of glucose to the brain.[1-4] Work with your health care provider to keep track of your hemoglobin A1c level, which is a marker for prediabetes. Ways to prevent diabetes overlap with ways of keeping your heart healthy, including exercise, a healthy weight, and a heart-healthy diet. Overconsumption of alcohol is a risk factor for diabetes, but moderate consumption of alcohol (one glass of red wine per day or less) is part of the Mediterranean diet discussed above.

5. Proper nutrition is essential, and it is a must to work with your health care provider to treat any vitamin deficiencies,

especially of the B vitamins, because vitamin B deficiencies are known to cause nerve and brain damage.

6. Brain trauma, even if mild like a concussion, is a known risk factor for dementia, although not necessarily for Alzheimer disease.[19,20] Brain trauma occurs most often in car accidents, household accidents (falling off a ladder, for example), sports injuries, and interpersonal conflict. Wearing a seat belt in the car is a simple and easy way to make brain injury less likely. Wearing a helmet when bicycling, riding a motorcycle, skiing, skateboarding, and participating in contact sports is another way to prevent brain injury. Use safety equipment and exercise caution when working around the house.

POSSIBLE WAYS TO REDUCE DEMENTIA RISK

1. Be careful when considering nutritional supplements. Studies are continuing, but so far it is not clear whether vitamins or fatty acid supplements help lower dementia risk.[14-18] There is promising evidence that vitamin E may help prevent dementia; however, too much vitamin E could increase the risk of prostate cancer.[15-17] Some studies suggest that vitamins C and D may be helpful. Apart from vitamin E, supplements do not seem to be harmful. Discuss any supplements you are considering with your health care provider because harmful interactions can occur with other medicines you take.

2. Lower levels of education have been associated with increased risk of Alzheimer disease, but it may simply mean that people with lower education have fewer resources for healthy living.[1-4] There is also evidence that this effect goes away when

more than one test is used to screen for memory problems in Alzheimer disease.[21] Still, it is never too late to learn new things or educate yourself. You can make taking a class at a local college or community center, enrolling in an online course, or even learning a new craft part of your self-care.

3. Exercise your brain as well as your body. Cognitive exercise and brain training have been shown to benefit cognition in people with and without Alzheimer disease, although this benefit is not specific to a particular activity or to long-term memory.[22-25] Examples of cognitive exercise include crossword and jigsaw puzzles, sudoku, word and image searches, memory and logic games, and more. The key is to keep your brain active with hobbies and activities that require you to think and solve problems. Researchers have found that three sessions per week lasting 30 to 60 minutes each have the most benefit.[22]

4. As you've learned by now, sensory stimulation is great for learning. You can even try the Dementia Connection Model for brain health! Exercise is multisensory. The auditory stimulation of music is known to promote cognition (see chapters 3–8). Many cognitive training exercises engage your hands, promoting tactile stimulation. Knitting, crocheting, and sewing; cooking and baking; and arts, crafts, and handiwork also engage multiple senses. Essential oils provide olfactory stimulation; consider using turmeric, frankincense, or rosemary oils.[26-29] I've shared throughout this book that many forms of sensory stimulation may slow Alzheimer disease, so hopefully the potential preventive actions are not a surprise. The beauty of it is that as you do these things with your loved one, you may be benefitting and protecting your own brain health too. Win-win!

5. Social interaction is another way to get sensory stimulation, and such approaches are currently under study for their potential in dementia prevention.[30,31] Simply put, talking and engaging with others requires cognition and sensory stimulation whether you are talking on the phone (auditory), knitting together in a group (visual and tactile), or sitting together outside chatting while you hear the birds sing (visual and auditory). Additionally, staying actively connected with friends, family, and your community helps to improve mood. Have you heard the saying "Happier people live longer"?

6. There is growing evidence that healthy sleep—getting an average of seven to eight hours each and every night—is associated with a lower risk of Alzheimer disease.[32,33] Try to have a consistent bedtime and waketime, and dedicate the place where you sleep to comfort and rest. Talk to your health care provider if you experience any difficulty sleeping (insomnia) or daytime tiredness. As a caregiver, you may also find that healthy and sufficient sleep makes everything you do just a little bit easier.

WHAT DOESN'T CURE OR PREVENT ALZHEIMER DISEASE

As I finish writing this book, I am saddened to say that there is no cure for Alzheimer disease nor any treatment that is guaranteed to prevent it. Consider that 5 million people in the United States live with the disease, with 16 million Americans providing unpaid caregiving. In total, the cost of paid and unpaid caregiving is estimated to be $516 billion per year.[1]

With a problem that large and costly, if a cure or prevention were proven, it would become widespread knowledge very quickly.

Be careful when considering anything claiming to be *the* cure or *the* prevention. Be especially wary if the treatment will add a large expense to your budget. This doesn't mean not trying the lifestyle changes shared in this chapter or not trying other things that you come across. It does mean being cautious and careful. Talk to your doctor about any supplements you consider taking, remembering that some dietary supplements might affect any medications you take. Consult your doctor about changing your diet or starting a new exercise program. You are looking after others—look after yourself, too, by asking your health care team to partner with you in a program of heart and brain health that works for you.

PUTTING IT INTO ACTION

Once you know what you can do to reduce your risk, the next step is to figure how to implement these strategies into your lifestyle. Once again, you can use the worksheet below. In the first column, write down an aspect of your life that could be healthier (for example, healthier diet or better sleep). Then write down the things you will try to improve that aspect of your health. After you have made that change for 30 days, put a checkmark or an X to record whether it worked for you. I recommend starting with one lifestyle choice and doing it for at least 30 days. You can really only master one strategy, one change, at a time. Own it and do it! Be sure that each change you make is intentional, just like your interactions with the one you are caring for. It takes four to six weeks to create a habit, even a healthy one. Then add another strategy for 30 days. As with the strategies you tried for your loved one, not everything you try for yourself will succeed. Keep trying and build your toolbox! There are many ways to care for your body, your heart, and your brain.

Health Concern	Strategy Used	1st Attempt	2nd Attempt	3rd Attempt	Outcome
Difficulty sleeping	Diffusing lavender at night	X	✓	✓	Will continue
	Journaling before bed	✓	✓	✓	Will continue

Note: A checkmark means the intervention was successful; an X indicates that it was not.

Challenge	Strategy Used	1st Attempt	2nd Attempt	3rd Attempt	Outcome

References

Chapter 1. What Is Alzheimer Disease?

1. Kraepelin, E. *Psychiatrie*, 8th ed. Vol. 1, *Allgemeine Psychiatrie*. Vol. 2, *Klinische Psychiatrie*. Leipzig: Barth, 1909–1910.
2. Jack, Clifford R., Jr., David A. Bennett, Kaj Blennow, et al. "NIA-AA Research Framework: Toward a Biological Definition of Alzheimer's Disease." *Alzheimer's and Dementia: The Journal of the Alzheimer's Association* 14, no. 4 (2018): 535–562. https://doi.org/doi:10.1016/j.jalz.2018.02.018.
3. Veerabhadrappa, Bhavana, Constance Delaby, Christophe Hirtz, et al. "Detection of Amyloid Beta Peptides in Body Fluids for the Diagnosis of Alzheimer's Disease: Where Do We Stand?" *Critical Reviews in Clinical Laboratory Sciences* 57, no. 2 (2019): 99–113. https://doi.org/doi:10.1080/10408363.2019.1678011.
4. Lane, C. A., J. Hardy, and J. M. Schott. "Alzheimer's Disease." *European Journal of Neurology* 25, no. 1 (2018): 59–70. https://doi.org/doi:10.1111/ene.13439.
5. "2020 Alzheimer's Disease Facts and Figures." *Alzheimer's and Dementia: The Journal of the Alzheimer's Association* 10 (2020): 1002/alz.12068. https://doi.org/doi:10.1002/alz.12068.
6. Karran, Eric, and Bart De Strooper. "The Amyloid Cascade Hypothesis: Are We Poised for Success or Failure?" Supplement, *Journal of Neurochemistry* 139, no. 2 (2016): 237–252. https://doi.org/doi: 10.1111/jnc.13632.
7. Crous-Bou, Marta, Carolina Minguillón, Nina Gramunt, and José Luis Molinuevo. "Alzheimer's Disease Prevention: From Risk Factors to Early Intervention." *Alzheimer's Research and Therapy* 9, no. 1 (2017): 71. https://doi.org/doi:10.1186/s13195-017-0297-z.
8. Van Erum, Jan, Debby Van Dam, and Peter Paul de Deyn. "Sleep and Alzheimer's Disease: A Pivotal Role for the Suprachiasmatic Nucleus." *Sleep Medicine Reviews* 40 (2018): 17–27. https://doi.org/doi:10.1016/j.smrv.2017.07.005.
9. Braak, Heiko, and Eva Braak. "Staging of Alzheimer's Disease-Related Neurofibrillary Changes." *Neurobiology of Aging* 16, no. 3

(1995): 271–278; discussion, 278–284. https://doi.org/doi:10
.1016/0197-4580(95)00021-6.

Chapter 2. What Is the Dementia Connection Model?

1. Reisberg, Barry, Sunnie Kenowsky, Emile H. Franssen, Stefanie R. Auer, and Liduin E. M. Souren. "Towards a Science of Alzheimer's Disease Management: A Model Based upon Current Knowledge of Retrogenesis." *International Psychogeriatrics* 11, no.1 (1999): 7–23. https://doi.org/doi:10.1017/s1041610299005554.
2. Hirono, N., E. Mori, Y. Ikejiri, et al. "Procedural Memory in Patients with Mild Alzheimer's Disease." *Dementia and Geriatric Cognitive Disorders* 8, no. 4 (1997): 210–216.
3. Freitas, Joshua J. *The Dementia Concept.* Raleigh, NC: Regal House, 2015.

Chapter 3. Using the Dementia Connection Model

1. Masika, Golden M., Yu S. F. Doris, and Polly W. C. Li. "Visual Art Therapy as a Treatment Option for Cognitive Decline among Older Adults: A Systematic Review and Meta-Analysis." *Journal of Advanced Nursing* (March 23, 2020). https://doi.org/doi:10.1111 /jan.14362.
2. "Art and Music." Alzheimer's Association website. Accessed April 6, 2020. https://alz.org/help-support/caregiving/daily-care /art-music.
3. Adams, Francis M., and Charles E. Osgood. "A Cross-Cultural Study of the Affective Meanings of Color." *Journal of Cross-Cultural Psychology* 4 (1973): 135–157. https://doi.org/doi:10.1177 /002202217300400201.
4. Dunne, Tracy E., Sandy A. Neargarder, P. B. Cipolloni, and Alice Cronin-Golomb. "Visual Contrast Enhances Food and Liquid Intake in Advanced Alzheimer's Disease." *Clinical Nutrition* 23, no. 4 (2004): 533–538.
5. Freitas, Joshua J. *The Dementia Concept.* Raleigh, NC: Regal House, 2015.
6. Koelsch, Stefan. "Brain Correlates of Music-Evoked Emotions." *Nature Reviews Neuroscience* 15, no. 3 (2014): 170–180. https:// doi.org/doi:10.1038/nrn3666.

7. King, J. B., K. G. Jones, E. Goldberg, et al. "Increased Functional Connectivity after Listening to Favored Music in Adults with Alzheimer Dementia." *Journal of Prevention of Alzheimer's Disease* 6, no. 1 (2019): 56–62. https://doi.org/doi:10.14283/jpad.2018.19.

8. Fang, Rong, Shengxuan Ye, Jiangtao Huangfu, and David P. Calimag. "Music Therapy Is a Potential Intervention for Cognition of Alzheimer's Disease: A Mini-Review." *Translational Neurodegeneration* 6 (2017): 2. https://doi.org/doi:10.1186/s40035-017 -0073-9.

9. Rossato-Bennett, Michael, dir. *Alive Inside: A Story of Music and Memory*. New York: Projector Media, 2014.

10. Dayawansa, Samantha, Katsumi Umeno, and Hiromasa Takakura. "Autonomic Responses during Inhalation of Natural Fragrance of Cedrol in Humans." *Autonomic Neuroscience: Basic and Clinical* 108, no. 1–2 (2003): 79–86. https://doi.org/doi:10.1016/j.autneu .2003.08.002.

11. Jager, W., G. Buchbauer, L. Jirovetz, and M. Fritzer. "Percutaneous Absorption of Lavender Oil from a Massage Oil." *Journal of the Society for Cosmetic Chemistry* 43 (1992): 49–54.

12. Benny, Anju, and Jayu Thomas. "Essential Oils as Treatment Strategy for Alzheimer's Disease: Current and Future Perspectives." *Planta Medica* 85, no. 3 (2019): 239–248. https://doi.org /doi:10.1055/a-0758-0188.

13. Aromatic Plant Research Center website. Accessed April 6, 2020. https://aromaticplant.org.

14. Atsumi, Toshiko, and Keiichi Tonosaki. "Smelling Lavender and Rosemary Increases Free Radical Scavenging Activity and Decreases Cortisol Level in Saliva." *Psychiatry Research* 150, no. 1 (2007): 89–96. https://doi.org/10.1016/j.psychres.2005 .12.012.

15. Ayaz, Muhammad, Abdul Sadiq, Muhammad Juniad, et al. "Neuroprotective and Anti-Aging Potentials of Essential Oils from Aromatic and Medicinal Plants." *Frontiers in Aging Neuroscience* 9 (2017): 168. https://doi.org/doi:10.3389/fnagi.2017 .00168.

16. McCaffrey, Ruth, Debra J. Thomas, and Ann Orth Kinzelman. "The Effects of Lavender and Rosemary Essential Oils on Test-Taking Anxiety among Graduate Nursing Students." *Holistic*

Nursing Practice 23, no. 2 (2009): 88–93. https://doi.org/doi:10 .1097/HNP.0b013e3181a110aa.

17. Banks, Duncan. "What Is Brain Plasticity and Why Is It So Important?" The Conversation. Accessed April 6, 2020. http:// theconversation.com/what-is-brain-plasticity-and-why-is-it-so -important-55967.

18. Tsalamlal, Yacine, Michele-Ange Amorim, Jean-Claude Martin, and Mehdi Ammi. "Modeling Emotional Valence Integration from Voice and Touch." *Frontiers in Psychology* 9 (2018): 1966. https://doi.org/doi:10.3389/fpsyg.2018.01966.

19. Barreto, Philipe de Souto, Julien Delrieu, Sandrine Andrieu, Bruno Vellas, and Yves Rolland. "Physical Activity and Cognitive Function in Middle-Aged and Older Adults: An Analysis of 104,909 People from 20 Countries." *Mayo Clinical Proceedings* 91, no. 11 (2016): 1515–1524. https:/doi.org/doi:10.1016/j .mayocp.2016.06.032.

20. Williams, Kristine, and Susan Kemper. "Exploring Interventions to Reduce Cognitive Decline in Aging." *Journal of Psychosocial Nursing and Mental Health Services* 48, no. 5 (2010): 42–51. https://doi.org/doi:10.3928/02793695-20100331-03.

21. Lautenschlager, Nicola T., Kay L. Cox, Leon Flicker, et al. "Effect of Physical Activity on Cognitive Function in Older Adults at Risk for Alzheimer's Disease." *Journal of American Medical Association* 300, no. 9 (2008): 1027–1037. https://doi.org/doi: 10.1001/jama.300.9.1027.

22. Fotuhi, Majid, David Do, and Clifford Jack. "Modifiable Factors That Alter the Size of the Hippocampus with Aging." *Nature Reviews Neurology* 8, no. 4 (2012): 189–202. https://doi.org/doi: 10.1038/nrneurol.2012.27.

23. Vann, Madeline R. "How Animal Therapy Helps Dementia Patients." Everyday Health. Last updated April 20, 2010. https:// www.everydayhealth.com/alzheimers/how-animal-therapy -helps-dementia-patients.aspx.

24. Sauer, Alisa. "Pros and Cons of Doll Therapy for Alzheimer's." Alzheimers.net, March 22, 2017. https://www.alzheimers.net /8-6-14-doll-therapy-alzheimers/.

25. Nierenberg, Cari. "The Science of Essential Oils: Does Using Scents Make Sense?" LiveScience.com, September 3, 2015.

https://www.livescience.com/52080-essential-oils-science
-health-effects.html.

Chapter 5. Eating, Feeding, and Nutrition Challenges

1. Freitas, Joshua J. *The Dementia Concept*. Raleigh, NC: Regal House, 2015.
2. Dunne, Tracy E., Sandy A. Neargarder, P. B. Cipolloni, and Alice Cronin-Golomb. "Visual Contrast Enhances Food and Liquid Intake in Advanced Alzheimer's Disease." *Clinical Nutrition* 23, no. 4 (2004): 533–538.
3. Adams, Francis M., and Charles E. Osgood. "A Cross-Cultural Study of the Affective Meanings of Color." *Journal of Cross-Cultural Psychology* 4 (1973): 135–157. https://doi.org/doi:10.1177 /002202217300400201.
4. McCaffrey, Ruth, Debra J. Thomas, and Ann Orth Kinzelman. "The Effects of Lavender and Rosemary Essential Oils on Test-Taking Anxiety among Graduate Nursing Students." *Holistic Nursing Practice* 23, no. 2 (2009): 88–93. https://doi.org/doi:10 .1097/HNP.0b013e3181a110aa.
5. Atsumi, Toshiko, and Keiichi Tonosaki. "Smelling Lavender and Rosemary Increases Free Radical Scavenging Activity and Decreases Cortisol Level in Saliva." *Psychiatry Research* 150, no. 1 (2007): 89–96. https://doi.org/10.1016/j.psychres.2005.12.012.
6. Snow, Teepa. "How Do We Safely Help Someone Transition from Moving to Sitting?" Positive Approach to Care. May 19, 2019. https://teepasnow.com/how-to-assist-someone-to-sit/.
7. McLeod, S. "Pavlov's Dogs." Simply Psychology. Accessed September 13, 2019. https://www.simplypsychology.org/pavlov.html.

Chapter 6. Sleeping Challenges

1. "Healthy Sleep Tips." National Sleep Foundation website. Accessed April 10, 2020. https://www.sleepfoundation.org /articles/healthy-sleep-tips.
2. Koulivand, Peir Hossein, Maryam Khaleghi Ghadiri, and Ali Gorji. "Lavender and the Nervous System." *Evidence-Based Complementary and Alternative Medicine* (2013): 681304. https://doi.org/doi: 10.1155/2013/681304.

3. Benny, Anju, and Jayu Thomas. "Essential Oils as Treatment Strategy for Alzheimer's Disease: Current and Future Perspectives." *Planta Medica* 85, no. 3 (2019): 239–248. https://doi.org /doi:10.1055/a-0758-0188.
4. Figueiro, Mariana G. "Light, Sleep and Circadian Rhythms in Older Adults with Alzheimer's Disease and Related Dementias." *Neurodegenerative Disease Management* 7, no. 2 (2017): 119–145. https://doi.org/doi:10.2217/nmt-2016-0060.
5. Hanford, Nicholas, and Mariana Figueiro. "Light Therapy and Alzheimer's Disease and Related Dementia: Past, Present, and Future." *Journal of Alzheimer's Disease* 33, no. 4 (2013): 913–922. https://doi.org/doi:10.3233/JAD-2012-121645.
6. Gonzalez-Lima, F. "Dose-Response Effects of Low-Level Light Therapy on Brain and Muscle." Presented at the 13th Annual International Conference on Dose-Response, Amherst, MA, April 23, 2014. https://cytonlabs.com/wp-content/uploads/2018/11 /Prof-GL-Dose-Reponse-LLLT-on-Brain-and-Muscle.pdf.

Chapter 7. Toileting Challenges

1. Al-Zubaidi, Taghreed Zuhair. "Towards a Dementia-Friendly Built Environment: Wayfinding Systems to Support Persons with Dementia in Geriatric Psychiatry Units." Master's thesis, Ontario College of Art and Design University, 2015. http://openresearch .ocadu.ca/id/eprint/1316/1/Zuhair%20Al-Zubaidi_Taghreed _2015_MDES_INCD_MRP.pdf.
2. "Dementia Friendly Print." *Solopress* (blog). November 10, 2014. https://www.solopress.com/blog/print-inspiration/dementia -friendly-print/.
3. "Water: How Much Should You Drink Every Day?" Mayo Clinic website, September 6, 2017. https://www.mayoclinic.org /healthy-lifestyle/nutrition-and-healthy-eating/in-depth/water /art-20044256.
4. Benny, Anju, and Jayu Thomas. "Essential Oils as Treatment Strategy for Alzheimer's Disease: Current and Future Perspectives." *Planta Medica* 85, no. 3 (2019): 239–248. https://doi.org /doi:10.1055/a-0758-0188.
5. Atsumi, Toshiko, and Keiichi Tonosaki. "Smelling Lavender and

Rosemary Increases Free Radical Scavenging Activity and Decreases Cortisol Level in Saliva." *Psychiatry Research* 150, no. 1 (2007): 89–96. https://doi.org/10.1016/j.psychres.2005.12.012.
6. McCaffrey, Ruth, Debra J. Thomas, and Ann Orth Kinzelman. "The Effects of Lavender and Rosemary Essential Oils on Test-Taking Anxiety among Graduate Nursing Students." *Holistic Nursing Practice* 23, no. 2 (2009): 88–93. https://doi.org/doi:10.1097/HNP.0b013e3181a110aa.

Chapter 9. Pain and Pain Management

1. Binnekade, Tarik T., Janime Van Kooten, Frank Lobbezoo, et al. "Pain Experience in Dementia Subtypes: A Systematic Review." *Current Alzheimer Research* 14, no. 5 (2017): 471–485. https://doi.org/doi:10.2174/1567205013666160602234109.
2. Achterberg, Wilco, Stefan Lautenbacher, Bettina Husebo, Ane Erdal, and Keela Herr. "Pain in Dementia." *Pain Reports* 5, no.1 (2019): e803. https://doi.org/doi:10.1097/PR9.0000000000000803.
3. Barry, Heather E., Carole Parsons, A. Peter Passmore, and Carmel M. Hughes. "Exploring the Prevalence of and Factors Associated with Pain: A Cross-Sectional Study of Community-Dwelling People with Dementia." *Health and Social Care in the Community* 24, no. 3 (2016): 270–282. https://doi.org/doi:10.1111/hsc.12204.
4. de Souto Barreto, Philipe, Julien Delrieu, Sandrine Andrieu, Bruno Vellas, and Yves Rolland. "Physical Activity and Cognitive Function in Middle-Aged and Older Adults: An Analysis of 104,909 People from 20 Countries." *Mayo Clinic Proceedings* 91, no. 11 (2016): 1515–1524. https://doi.org/doi:10.1016/j.mayocp.2016.06.032.
5. Guitar, Nicole A., Denise M. Connelly, Lindsay S. Nagamatsu, Joseph B. Orange, and Susan W. Muir-Hunter. "The Effects of Physical Exercise on Executive Function in Community-Dwelling Older Adults Living with Alzheimer's-Type Dementia: A Systematic Review." *Ageing Research Reviews* 47 (2018): 159–167. https://doi.org/doi:10.1016/j.arr.2018.07.009.
6. Lautenschlager, Nicola T., Kay L. Cox, Leon Flicker, et al. "Effect of Physical Activity on Cognitive Function in Older Adults at Risk

for Alzheimer Disease: A Randomized Trial." *Journal of the American Medical Association* 300, no. 9 (2008): 1027–1037. https:// doi.org/doi:10.1001/jama.300.9.1027.

Chapter 10. Depression, Hallucinations, and Delusions

1. Lautenschlager, Nicola T., Kay L. Cox, and Kathryn A. Ellis. "Physical Activity for Cognitive Health: What Advice Can We Give to Older Adults with Subjective Cognitive Decline and Mild Cognitive Impairment?" *Dialogues in Clinical Neuroscience* 21, no. 1 (2019): 61–68.
2. Jia, Rui-Xia, Jing-Hong Liang, Yong Xu, and Ying-Quan Wang. "Effects of Physical Activity and Exercise on the Cognitive Function of Patients with Alzheimer Disease: A Meta-Analysis." *BMC Geriatrics* 19, no. 1 (2019): 181. https://doi.org/doi:10 .1186/s12877-019-1175-2.
3. Choi, Karmel W., Chia-Yen Chen, Murray B. Stein, et al. "Major Depressive Disorder Working Group of the Psychiatric Genomics Consortium. Assessment of Bidirectional Relationships between Physical Activity and Depression among Adults: A 2-Sample Mendelian Randomization Study." *JAMA Psychiatry* 76, no. 4 (2019): 399–408. https://doi.org/10.1001/jamapsychiatry.2018 .4175.
4. Paul Natalie, Carol Lotter, and Werdie van Staden. "Patient Reflections on Individual Music Therapy for a Major Depressive Disorder or Acute Phase Schizophrenia Spectrum Disorder." *Journal of Music Therapy* (2020): thaa001. https://doi.org/doi:10.1093 /jmt/thaa001.
5. Fang Rong, Shengxuan Ye, Jiangtao Huangfu, and David P. Calimag. "Music Therapy Is a Potential Intervention for Cognition of Alzheimer's Disease: A Mini-Review." *Translational Neurodegeneration* 6 (2017): 2. https://doi.org/doi:10.1186/s40035-017-0073-9.
6. Rossato-Bennett, Michael, dir. *Alive Inside: A Story of Music and Memory*. New York: Projector Media, 2014.
7. Pongan, Elodie, Barbara Tillmann, Yohana Leveque, et al. "Can Musical or Painting Interventions Improve Chronic Pain, Mood, Quality of Life, and Cognition in Patients with Mild Alzheimer's Disease? Evidence from a Randomized Controlled Trial." *Journal*

of Alzheimer's Disease 60, no. 2 (2017): 663–677. https://doi.org
/doi:10.3233/JAD-170410.

8. Masika, Golden M., Yu S. F. Doris, and Polly W. C. Li. "Visual Art
Therapy as a Treatment Option for Cognitive Decline among
Older Adults: A Systematic Review and Meta-Analysis." *Journal of
Advanced Nursing* (March 23, 2020). https://doi.org/doi:10.1111
/jan.14362.

9. Vann, Madeline R. "How Animal Therapy Helps Dementia Patients." Everyday Health, April 20, 2020. https://www.everyday
health.com/alzheimers/how-animal-therapy-helps-dementia
-patients.aspx.

10. Sauer, Alisa. "Pros and Cons of Doll Therapy for Alzheimer's."
Alzheimers.net, March 22, 2017. https://www.alzheimers.net
/8-6-14-doll-therapy-alzheimers/.

11. Xiong, Mei, Li Yanzhang, and Tang Ping. "Effectiveness of Aromatherapy Massage and Inhalation on Symptoms of Depression in
Chinese Community-Dwelling Older Adults." *Journal of Alternative and Complementary Medicine* 24, no. 7 (2018): 717–724.
https://doi.org/10.1089/acm.2017.0320.

Chapter 11. Repetitive Behavior, Rummaging, and Collecting

1. "Repetitive Behaviors." UCLA Alzheimer's and Dementia Care
Program website. Accessed April 20, 2020. https://www
.uclahealth.org/dementia/repetitive-behaviors.

2. "Help and Support: Stages and Behaviors—Repetition." Alzheimer's
Association website. Accessed April 20, 2020. https://www.alz
.org/help-support/caregiving/stages-behaviors/repetition.

3. Vann, Madeline. "How Animal Therapy Helps Dementia Patients."
Everyday Health. Last updated April 20, 2010. https://www
.everydayhealth.com/alzheimers/how-animal-therapy-helps
-dementia-patients.aspx.

4. Freitas, Joshua J. *The Dementia Concept.* Raleigh, NC: Regal House,
2015.

5. Atsumi, Toshiko, and Keiichi Tonosaki. "Smelling Lavender and
Rosemary Increases Free Radical Scavenging Activity and Decreases Cortisol Level in Saliva." *Psychiatry Research* 150, no. 1
(2007): 89–96. https://doi.org/10.1016/j.psychres.2005.12.012.

6. McCaffrey, Ruth, Debra J. Thomas, and Ann Orth Kinzelman. "The Effects of Lavender and Rosemary Essential Oils on Test-Taking Anxiety among Graduate Nursing Students." *Holistic Nursing Practice* 23, no. 2 (2009): 88–93. https://doi.org/doi:10.1097/HNP.0b013e3181a110aa.

Chapter 12. Sundowning, Aggression, and Wandering

1. Atsumi, Toshiko, and Keiichi Tonosaki. "Smelling Lavender and Rosemary Increases Free Radical Scavenging Activity and Decreases Cortisol Level in Saliva." *Psychiatry Research* 150, no. 1 (2007): 89–96. https://doi.org/10.1016/j.psychres.2005.12.012.
2. McCaffrey, Ruth, Debra J. Thomas, and Ann Orth Kinzelman. "The Effects of Lavender and Rosemary Essential Oils on Test-Taking Anxiety among Graduate Nursing Students." *Holistic Nursing Practice* 23, no. 2 (2009): 88–93. https://doi.org/doi:10.1097/HNP.0b013e3181a110aa.
3. Fang, Rong, Shengxuan Ye, Jiangtao Huangfu, and David P. Calimag. "Music Therapy Is a Potential Intervention for Cognition of Alzheimer's Disease: A Mini-Review." *Translational Neurodegeneration* 6 (2017): 2. https://doi.org/doi:10.1186/s40035-017-0073-9.
4. Rossato-Bennett, Michael, dir. *Alive Inside: A Story of Music and Memory*. New York: Projector Media, 2014.
5. Pongan, Elodie, Barbara Tillmann, Yohana Leveque, et al. "Can Musical or Painting Interventions Improve Chronic Pain, Mood, Quality of Life, and Cognition in Patients with Mild Alzheimer's Disease? Evidence from a Randomized Controlled Trial." *Journal of Alzheimer's Disease* 60, no. 2 (2017): 663–677. https://doi.org/doi:10.3233/JAD-170410.
6. Vann, Madeline. "How Animal Therapy Helps Dementia Patients." Everyday Health. Last updated April 20, 2010. https://www.everydayhealth.com/alzheimers/how-animal-therapy-helps-dementia-patients.aspx.
7. Neal, Martin, and Philip Barton Wright. "Validation Therapy for Dementia." *Cochrane Database of Systematic Reviews* 3 (2003): CD001394. https://doi.org/10.1002/14651858.CD001394.

Chapter 13. Intentional Care

1. "Depression: What Is Burnout?" InformedHealth.org. Last updated June 18, 2020. https://www.ncbi.nlm.nih.gov/books /NBK279286/.
2. Yang, Fang, Mao Ran, and Wei Luo. "Depression of Persons with Dementia and Family Caregiver Burden: Finding Positives in Caregiving as a Moderator." *Geriatrics and Gerontology International* 19, no. 5 (2019): 414–418. https://doi.org/10.1111/ggi .13632.

Chapter 14. Promoting Brain Health

1. Alzheimer's Association. *2020 Alzheimer's Disease Facts and Figures*. Chicago: Alzheimer's Association, 2020. https://www.alz .org/media/Documents/alzheimers-facts-and-figures_1.pdf.
2. Phillips, Cristy, Mehmet Akif Bakti, Devsmita Das, Bill Lin, and Ahmad Salehi. "The Link between Physical Activity and Cognitive Dysfunction in Alzheimer Disease." *Physical Therapy* 95, no. 7 (2015): 1046–1060. https://doi.org/doi:10.2522/ptj .20140212.
3. Williams, Kristine N., and Susan Kemper. "Interventions to Reduce Cognitive Decline in Aging." *Journal of Psychosocial Nursing and Mental Health Services* 48, no. 5 (2010): 42–51. https://doi.org/10.3928/02793695-20100331-03.
4. Lipnicki, Darren M., Steve R. Makkar, John D. Crawford, et al. "Determinants of Cognitive Performance and Decline in 20 Diverse Ethno-Regional Groups: A COSMIC Collaboration Cohort Study." *PLOS Medicine* 16, no. 7 (2019): e1002853. https://doi.org/10.1371/journal.pmed.1002853.
5. "8 Things You Can Do to Prevent Heart Disease and Stroke." American Heart Association, March 14, 2019. https://www.heart.org /en/healthy-living/healthy-lifestyle/prevent-heart-disease-and -stroke.
6. Xu, Wei, Hui Fu Wang, Yu Wan, Chen-Chen Tan, Jin-Tai Yu, and Lan Tan. "Leisure Time Physical Activity and Dementia Risk: A Dose-Response Meta-Analysis of Prospective Studies." *BMJ Open* 7, no. 10 (2017): e014706. https://doi.org/doi:10.1136 /bmjopen-2016-014706.

7. Tan, Zaldy S., Nicole L. Spartano, Alexa S. Beiser, et al. "Physical Activity, Brain Volume, and Dementia Risk: The Framingham Study." *Journals of Gerontology: Series A, Biological Sciences and Medical Sciences* 72, no. 6 (2017): 789–795. https://doi.org/10.1093/gerona/glw130.

8. Stephen, Ruth, Kristiina Hongisto, Alina Solomon, and Eija Lönnroos. "Physical Activity and Alzheimer's Disease: A Systematic Review." *Journals of Gerontology: Series A, Biological Sciences and Medical Sciences* 72, no. 6 (2017): 733–739. https://doi.org/doi:10.1093/gerona/glw251.

9. Jia, Rui-Xia, Jing-Hong Liang, Yong Xu, and Ying-Quan Wang. "Effects of Physical Activity and Exercise on the Cognitive Function of Patients with Alzheimer Disease: A Meta-Analysis." *BMC Geriatrics* 19, no. 1 (2019): 181. https://doi.org/doi:10.1186/s12877-019-1175-2.

10. Daimiel, Lidia, Miguel A. Martínez-González, Dolores Corella, et al. "Physical Fitness and Physical Activity Association with Cognitive Function and Quality of Life: Baseline Cross-Sectional Analysis of the PREDIMED-Plus Trial." *Scientific Reports* 10, no. 1 (2020): 3472. https://doi.org/doi:10.1038/s41598-020-59458-6.

11. US Department of Health and Human Services. *Physical Activity Guidelines for Americans.* 2nd ed. Washington, DC: US Department of Health and Human Services, 2019. https://health.gov/sites/default/files/2019-09/Physical_Activity_Guidelines_2nd_edition.pdf.

12. Valls-Pedret, Cinta, Aleix Sala-Vila, Mercè Serra-Mir, et al. "Mediterranean Diet and Age-Related Cognitive Decline: A Randomized Clinical Trial." *JAMA Internal Medicine* 175, no. 7 (2015): 1094–1103. https://doi.org/doi:10.1001/jamainternmed.2015.1668.

13. Petersson, Sara Danuta, and Elena Philippou. "Mediterranean Diet, Cognitive Function, and Dementia: A Systematic Review of the Evidence." *Advances in Nutrition* 7, no. 5 (2016): 889–904. htpps://doi.org/doi:10.3945/an.116.012138.

14. Chen, Xi, Brook Maguire, Henry Brodaty, and Fiona O'Leary. "Dietary Patterns and Cognitive Health in Older Adults: A Systematic Review." *Journal of Alzheimer's Disease* 67, no. 2 (2019): 583–619. https://doi.org/doi:10.3233/JAD-180468.

15. Rutjes, Anne Ws, David A. Denton, Marcello Di Nisio, et al. "Vitamin and Mineral Supplementation for Maintaining Cognitive Function in Cognitively Healthy People in Mid and Late Life." *Cochrane Database Systematic Reviews* 12, no. 12 (2019): CD011906. https://doi.org/doi:10.1002/14651858.CD011906 .pub2.

16. McCleery, Jenny, Rajesh P. Abraham, David A. Denton, et al. "Vitamin and Mineral Supplementation for Preventing Dementia or Delaying Cognitive Decline in People with Mild Cognitive Impairment." *Cochrane Database of Systematic Reviews* 11, no. 11 (2018): CD011905. https://doi.org./doi:10.1002/14651858 .CD011905.pub2.

17. Farina, N., D. Llewellyn, M. G. Isaac, and N. Tabet. "Vitamin E for Alzheimer's Dementia and Mild Cognitive Impairment." *Cochrane Database of Systematic Reviews* 1, no. 1 (2017): CD002854. https://doi.org/doi:10.1002/14651858.CD002854.pub4.

18. Burckhardt, Marion, Max Herke, Tobias Wustmann, Stefan Watzke, Gero Langer, and Astrid Fink. "Omega-3 Fatty Acids for the Treatment of Dementia." *Cochrane Database of Systematic Reviews* 4, no. 4 (2016): CD009002. https://doi.org/doi:10.1002 /14651858.CD009002.pub3.

19. Mollayeva, Tatyana, Shirin Mollayeva, Nicole Pacheco, Andrea D'Souza, and Angela Colantonio. "The Course and Prognostic Factors of Cognitive Outcomes after Traumatic Brain Injury: A Systematic Review and Meta-Analysis." *Neuroscience and Biobehavioral Reviews* 99 (2019): 198–250. https://doi.org/10.1016 /j.neubiorev.2019.01.011.

20. Huang, Chi-Hsien, Chi-Wei Lin, Yi-Che Lee, et al. "Is Traumatic Brain Injury a Risk Factor for Neurodegeneration? A Meta-Analysis of Population-Based Studies." *BMC Neurology* 18, no. 1 (2018): 184. https://doi.org/doi:10.1186/s12883-018-1187-0.

21. Ranson, Janice M., Elżbieta Kuźma, William Hamilton, Graciela Muniz-Terrera, Kenneth M. Langa, and David J. Llewellyn. "Predictors of Dementia Misclassification when Using Brief Cognitive Assessments." *Neurology in Clinical Practice* 9, no. 2 (2019): 109–117. https://doi.org/doi:10.1212/CPJ.0000000000000566.

22. Lampit, Amit, Harry Hallock, and Michael Valenzuela. "Computerized Cognitive Training in Cognitively Healthy Older Adults:

A Systematic Review and Meta-Analysis of Effect Modifiers."
PLOS Medicine 11, no. 11 (2014): e10011756. https://doi.org/10
.1371/journal.pmed.1001756.

23. Martin, Mike, Linda Clare, Anne Mareike Altgassen, Michelle H.
Cameron, and Franzisca Zehnder. "Cognition-Based Interven-
tions for Healthy Older People and People with Mild Cognitive
Impairment." *Cochrane Database of Systematic Reviews* 19,
no. 1 (2011): CD006220. https://doi.org/10.1002/14651858
.CD006220.pub2.

24. Gates, Nicola J., Robin W. M. Vernooij, Marcello Di Nisio, et al.
"Computerised Cognitive Training for Preventing Dementia in
People with Mild Cognitive Impairment." *Cochrane Database of
Systematic Reviews* 3, no. 3 (2019): CD012279. https://doi.org/10
.1002/14651858.CD012279.pub2.

25. Bahar-Fuchs, Alex, Anthony Martyr, Anita My Goh, Julieta Sa-
bates, and Linda Clare. "Cognitive Training for People with Mild
to Moderate Dementia." *Cochrane Database of Systematic Reviews*
3, no. 3 (2019): CD013069. https://doi.org/10.1002/14651858
.CD013069.pub2.

26. Atsumi, Toshiko, and Keiichi Tonosaki. "Smelling Lavender and
Rosemary Increases Free Radical Scavenging Activity and Decreases Cortisol Level in Saliva." *Psychiatry Research* 150, no. 1
(2007): 89–96.

27. Dayawansa, Samantha, Katsumi Umeno, and Hiromasa Takakura.
"Autonomic Responses During Inhalation of Natural Fragrance
of Cedrol in Humans." *Autonomic Neuroscience: Basic and Clinical*
108, no. 1–2 (2003): 79–86. https://doi.org/doi:10.1016/j.autneu
.2003.08.002.

28. Benny, Anju, and Jayu Thomas. "Essential Oils as Treatment Strategy for Alzheimer's Disease: Current and Future Perspectives."
Planta Medica 85, no. 3 (2019): 239–248. https://doi.org/doi:10
.1055/a-0758-0188.

29. Ayaz, Muhammad, Abdul Sadiq, Muhammad Junaid, Farhat
Ullah, Fazal Subhan, and Jawad Ahmed. "Neuroprotective and
Anti-Aging Potentials of Essential Oils from Aromatic and
Medicinal Plants." *Frontiers in Aging Neuroscience* 9, no. 168
(2017): 168. https://doi.org/doi:10.3389/fnagi.2017.00168.

30. Penninkilampi, Ross, Anne-Nicole Casey, Maria Fiatarone Singh, and Henry Brodaty. "The Association between Social Engagement, Loneliness, and Risk of Dementia: A Systematic Review and Meta-Analysis." *Journal of Alzheimer's Disease* 66, no. 4 (2018): 1619–1633. https://doi.org/10.3233/JAD-180439.

31. Sajeev, Gautam, Jennifer Weuve, John W. Jackson, et al. "Late-Life Cognitive Activity and Dementia: A Systematic Review and Bias Analysis." *Epidemiology* 27, no. 5 (2016): 732–742. doi:10.1097/EDE.0000000000000513.

32. Shi, Le, Si-Jing Chen, Meng-Ying Ma, et al. "Sleep Disturbances Increase the Risk of Dementia: A Systematic Review and Meta-Analysis." *Sleep Medicine Reviews* 40 (2018): 4–16. https://doi.org/10.1016/j.smrv.2017.06.010.

33. Bubu, Omonigho M., Michael Brannick, James Mortimer, et al. "Sleep, Cognitive Impairment, and Alzheimer's Disease: A Systematic Review and Meta-Analysis." *Sleep* 40, no. 1 (2017): 10.1093/sleep/zsw032. https://doi.org/10.1093/sleep/zsw032.

Index

acetaminophen, 99, 100
acetylcholine, 4
affirmative sensory stimulation.
 See sensory stimulation /
 sensory-based knowledge
aggression, 2, 13, 45, 111; in caregivers, 136; pain expressed as,
 97–98; sundowning-related,
 123; tips for managing, 125–31
agitation, 14, 26, 33, 45, 52, 58, 62
alcohol use, 74, 136, 141, 143
Alive Inside (documentary), 33
Alzheimer, Alois, 2–3, 4
Alzheimer disease, 1–3; advanced,
 13, 20, 23, 56, 109; clinical
 picture, 1, 7–14; definition, 2;
 diagnosis, 3, 12; early onset, 6,
 9–11, 70; lack of a cure for,
 146–47; moderate-stage, 11–13,
 14, 56, 70, 109; as mortality
 cause, 6, 7; prevalence, 6–7, 146
Alzheimer's Association website,
 31, 112
American Academy of Sleep Medicine, 32, 100
American Psychiatric Association,
 *Diagnostic and Statistical
 Manual of Mental Disorders*, 2
amygdala, 9–10, 14, 33
amyloid hypothesis, 4–5
amyloid plaques, 2, 3–5
anger, 26, 32–33, 51, 99, 111, 126
animals: stuffed or animatronic,
 39–40; therapy, 39. *See also*
 pets
anticipation skills, 9, 48, 56

anxiety, 13, 14, 88, 90–91, 92, 97,
 101
anxiety reduction techniques, 33,
 34, 35, 48, 49, 107, 128; tactile
 stimulation, 36–37, 41, 46, 62,
 63, 73, 91, 92, 106, 117, 127
APOE genes, 3
appetite, 35, 62, 64, 99
aromatherapy, 33–36, 108. *See also*
 essential oils
Aromatic Plant Research Center
 (APRC), 34
art / art therapy, 30–31, 107
attention, 10
attention improvement techniques,
 31, 32, 35–36, 45, 61, 92, 107;
 tactile stimulation, 36–37, 41,
 48, 62–63, 73, 127
auditory hallucinations, 14
auditory stimulation, 26–27, 28,
 32–33, 107, 128; for bathing and
 showering, 89, 90; for bathroom breaks, 82–83; cooking as,
 37–38; during mealtimes, 59,
 64; overstimulation in, 43–44;
 with pets and other animals, 39;
 for sleep environment, 72, 73.
 See also praise

baking and cooking, 37–39, 109,
 145
balance training, 142
bathing and showering, 48, 73,
 87–95
bathroom breaks, 51, 82–83, 127
Baun, Mara M., 39

bedtime, 124; routine for, 70, 71, 72–73, 75. *See also* sleep
behaviors, 24; overt, 45, 51; repetitive, 115–21; sensory stimulation and, 28
belief systems, false, 111
beta-amyloid 42, 4–5
blankets, weighted, 117, 125
blood pressure control, 142
blood sugar control, 142
body language, 24, 27, 29–30, 43, 45, 46
body weight, healthy, 142
boredom, 51, 70–71, 126, 127
brain changes, Alzheimer disease–related, 2–5; atrophy, 4, 9–11, 14–15, 105; blood and oxygen supply, 141–42; in brain lobes, 9–10, 11; chemistry, 105; plasticity and, 36
brain health techniques, 8, 38, 141–49
brain imaging, 3–4
brain training, 145
brain trauma, 144
Buchbauer, Gerhard, 34–35
burnout, 136

caffeinated beverages, 74
calmness, 25; during bathing and showering, 88–89, 91; in caregivers, 26–27, 46, 59, 117, 127, 135; environmental, 50; mimicking, 26–27, 46, 117; sensory-stimulation techniques for, 26–27, 32, 47, 72, 106, 118, 125, 128; for sleep promotion, 72, 74
caregivers: burnout, 136; calmness in, 26–27, 46, 59, 117, 127, 135; expectations, 21–22; frustration, 21, 22, 127; implications of retrogenesis for, 21–22; intentional interactions, 28, 147–48; mood, 30, 59, 74, 127; self-care, 133–36; support systems, 111–12, 136
caregiver strategies toolbox, 133; aggression, 129–31; bathing and showering, 93–95; brain health, 147–49; communication/language, 52–54; depression, 112–14; eating and nutrition, 64–67; repetitive behaviors, 119–21; self-care, 137–39; sleep challenges, 75–77; toileting, 84–86
caregiving, cost of, 146–47
choices, predetermined, 127
choking hazards, 37
cholesterol levels, 7, 142
circadian rhythm, 124
clinical picture, of Alzheimer disease, 1, 7–14
cognitive impairment: mild (MCI), 7–9; sleep patterns and, 71; toileting and, 79, 82; understimulation-related, 71
cognitive improvement/stimulation techniques, 33, 36, 37, 41, 100, 107, 108, 141, 145
collecting behavior, 115, 118
coloring activities, 107
colors, 12, 31–32, 44, 61, 80, 81, 90, 118
comfort objects, 72, 73. *See also* animals; dolls / doll therapy; pets
communication challenges, 43–54, 126; retrogenesis and, 19, 21, 43–45, 52. *See also* language

deficits; nonverbal communication; verbal communication
compassion, 129, 133
concentration impairment, 10, 91
concentration improvement techniques, 62–63, 91, 92, 107; sensory stimulation / sensory-based knowledge, 32, 35, 36–37, 41, 48, 62, 83, 127
confusion, 2, 33, 79, 99, 123, 126; management techniques, 36–37, 48, 60–61, 63–64, 116, 126
cooking and baking, 37–39, 109, 145
counseling, 108
crying, 45, 47, 51, 99

decision making, 57; with predetermined choices, 127
delusions, 109–12, 126
dementia, 5, 6; frontotemporal, 5; with Lewy bodies, 5; methods to reduce risk, 5, 7, 141–50; symptoms, 6; vascular, 5, 142
Dementia Concept, The (Freitas), 36
Dementia Connection Model, 1, 2, 17–28; for brain health, 145; definition, 17; in practice, 26–27; three R's (routine, remind, reward), 27, 51, 52, 60, 64, 71, 89, 124, 125. *See also* habilitation; retrogenesis; sensory stimulation / sensory-based knowledge
dental issues, 45, 51, 61, 64
depression, 75, 101, 105–9, 128
developmental age, 20–21, 23, 25, 27
diabetes, 7, 141, 143

diet, heart- and brain-healthy, 5, 142–44, 147
dolls / doll therapy, 40–41, 72, 108, 117, 120, 125
drug treatment, for Alzheimer disease, 4–5
drug use, 141

eating skills development, 17–19
eating skills impairment, 13, 23, 55–67, 75; assisted feeding and, 56, 57, 60, 62–63; retrogenesis and, 17–19, 22, 23, 55–58; tips for managing, 58–64
educational level, dementia risk and, 141, 144–45
embarrassment, 79, 88
emotional needs, 51, 52
emotions / emotional expression, 9–10, 13, 14, 19, 21, 34, 97; in caregivers, 135; habilitation and, 25–27; positive and negative, 24–25, 28, 89, 115; sensory stimulation / sensory-based knowledge effects, 25–27, 30, 31–33; validation, 49, 129. *See also specific emotions*
endorphins, 107
entorhinal cortex, 9–10
environment: in bathrooms, 80–82, 90–91; calm, 50; during meals, 56, 57, 58–60, 64; for sleeping, 71–72
essential oils, 26, 33–36, 62, 64, 112, 113; allergic reactions, 36, 90; application, 108, 128; calming effects, 128–29; citrus, 62, 66, 90, 108, 113, 138; frankincense, 100, 145; lavender, 72, 74, 76, 90, 117, 120, 125, 128–29,

essential oils (*cont.*)
130, 149; peppermint, 35, 83,
90, 100; Roman chamomile, 117;
rosemary, 83, 100, 117, 125, 145;
turmeric, 100, 145
executive brain functions, 9, 11,
48, 60
exercise: aerobic, 73–74, 142; for
aggression control, 128; for anxiety control, 128; cognitive, 145;
for dementia risk reduction, 5,
142, 147; for depression control,
107, 128, 197; lack of, 141; multisensory nature, 145; for pain
management, 100; as sensory
stimulation, 107; for sleep promotion, 73–74; timing, 73–74,
124; for tiredness control, 128;
for wandering control, 128
eye contact, 29, 46

facial expressions, 24, 27, 43, 45
falls, 12, 30, 69, 82, 90–91
false beliefs, 13
fear, 13, 46, 51, 88, 90–91, 127, 128
fear management techniques,
36–37, 41, 48, 62–63, 73, 91,
92, 107
fecal incontinence, 13
fight-or-flight response, 14,
125–26, 129
fluid intake, 82, 85
food: colors, flavors, and smell,
61–62; as distraction from
repetitive behaviors, 117; emotional response to, 25; increased
consumption, 31; as stimulant,
74
frontal lobe atrophy, 9–11, 56
frustration, 21, 22, 51, 111, 127

gene testing, 3
goodbyes, avoidance of, 128
grab bars, 82
grounding effect, 36–37
guilt, 105, 134, 138
gustatory stimulation, 25, 33,
37–38, 61–62, 73, 135

habilitation, 2, 22–27, 49; in
bathing and showering, 90, 92;
definition, 22–23; for eating
skills, 23, 60; sensory stimulation for, 45; for sleep promotion, 72–73; for sundowning
control, 124
hallucinations, 13, 14, 109–12, 126
hand gestures, 45, 46, 115, 116
hand-under-hand technique, 62,
63, 88, 91
happiness, 25, 27, 28, 29–30, 42,
146
hearing: brain regions involved in,
10, 11; effect on emotions, 25.
See also auditory stimulation
hearing problems, 11, 43–44, 47,
51
heart disease, risk factors, 141
heart health, 141–43
hippocampus, 9–10, 23, 33, 38
Hispanics, 6–7
hunger, 117, 127

ibuprofen, 100
incontinence, 13, 79, 82, 83, 84
incontinence products, 79, 84
independent skills deficits, 10–11
infections, 5, 51, 64, 82, 84
instructions, step-by-step approach,
47–48
intentional care, 133–39

International Classification of Disease, 2
irritability, 69, 70, 99, 123, 127

journaling, 138, 149
judgment deficits, 6, 11

language deficits, 6, 11, 19, 21, 45, 47; intervention strategies, 52–54
learning ability, 6, 23–24; procedural, 24, 25–26, 27. *See also* habilitation
light boxes, 124
lighting, 58, 59, 71–72, 73, 80, 90, 124
light therapy, 73, 113
limbic system, 9–10, 33–34, 37–38
living one's truth, 110–11
loneliness, 51
loved ones: deceased, 50, 105, 109, 111; forgetting names of, 11, 27, 111; separation from, 128

meals: environment during, 56, 57, 58–60, 64; scheduling of, 51. *See also* eating skills impairment
medical issues, 45, 50–51, 75, 84
medications, 64, 75, 84, 97–98, 99, 100
memories: questions about, 50; recollection of, 33, 37–38, 40; retrogenesis of, 12–13; sensory, 37–38
memory: brain regions responsible for, 10, 23; procedural, 23–24, 25, 60; short-term, 10, 12, 48
memory deficits, 2, 6; in mild cognitive impairment, 8, 9; in

moderate-stage Alzheimer disease, 11, 12–13; in normal aging, 8; progression, 9–10, 11; retrogenesis and, 17–22; short-term, 10, 12–13
metals exposure, as Alzheimer disease risk factor, 5
mimicking, 27, 30, 32, 46, 74, 117, 126
mobility impairment, 12, 19–20
mood, 10, 14; of caregivers, 30, 59, 74, 127; communication of, 46; effect of sensory stimulation on, 31–33, 37, 107; regulation of, 9–10
music: during bathing and showering, 90; effect on mood and emotions, 25, 32–33, 107, 112, 125, 128, 145; during exercise, 38; familiar songs, 89, 90; during mealtimes, 59, 64; for repetitive behavior control, 118; for sleep promotion, 72; for wandering control, 128

napping, 70–71, 100, 124
National Sleep Foundation, 71, 72
neurofibrillary tangles, 2, 3–5
neuroplasticity, 36
neurotransmitters, 4
nicotine, 74
nightlights, 71–72
nonverbal communication, 29–30; through art, 107; overt behavior as, 45; of pain, 97, 99; tips for improving, 46–47. *See also* sensory cues; verbal cues; visual cues
nutritional supplements, 144, 147

obsessions, 13
occupational therapy, 108
olfactory stimulation, 33–36, 117;
aromatherapy, 33–36, 108; for
bathing and showering, 90;
cooking as, 37–38; effect on
mood and emotions, 25,
26–27, 28, 117; during meals,
62; for sleep promotion, 72, 73.
See also essential oils
opioids, 99
orientation deficits, 6, 12
overstimulation, 41–42, 43–44,
50, 87–88, 115, 126, 127
overt behaviors, 45, 51

pain: assessment and treatment,
99–100; as contraindication to
bathing, 91; effect on eating
ability, 64; effect on sleep, 69,
74; expression of, 97–98; management, 74, 97–103; as repetitive behavior cause, 115, 117;
retrogenesis in, 97–98; during
toileting, 82
palliative care, 100
paranoia, 2, 14
parietal areas, of the brain, 12
"perfect day" method, 124–25
peripheral vision loss, 12, 46, 60,
62, 91
personality changes, 10, 21
personal names: forgetting of, 8,
11, 27; forms of, 44, 49
pesticides, as Alzheimer disease
risk factor, 5
pets, 39–40, 41, 70, 72, 108, 112,
117, 125, 128
physical activities, 38. See also
exercise

physical needs: as aggression
cause, 126, 127; communication
of, 51, 52; as eating deterrent,
59; as repetitive behavior cause,
115, 117; as wandering cause,
127
positive reinforcement, 64, 82–83,
89, 92. See also habilitation
praise, 46, 48, 49, 64, 82–83, 106,
108
problem-solving skills, 9, 56, 57,
87, 97
proteins, toxic, in Alzheimer disease pathology, 3–5, 14–15
psychological symptoms, 14
psychologists, 108

questions, asking: about memories,
50; open-ended, 49; repetitive,
117

reality, of persons with dementia,
50, 110–11
regression, 19, 117. See also retrogenesis; retroregression
Reisberg, Barry, 17, 20, 21
reminiscing, 50
repetitive behaviors, 115–21
rest periods, 124
retrogenesis, 2, 17–22, 25; aggression and, 125–26; of artistic
expression, 31; bathing/shower-
ing and, 87–89; of the brain,
105; in communication, 43–45,
52; in eating ability, 55–58; in
language use, 47; memory
deficits and, 17–22; in pain,
97–98; repetitive behaviors and,
115–16, 117; sleep and, 69–71;
sundowning and, 123–25; in

time perception, 12–13, 109, 111; in toileting, 79; wandering and, 125–26

retrogression, 19, 22, 45, 50, 61, 105, 109, 111, 117, 128. *See also* retrogenesis

reward, 27, 52, 58, 64, 71, 89, 124, 125

risk factors, for dementia, 7, 141; reduction methods, 5, 7, 141–50

routine, 51; for bathing and showering, 88–89; for bedtime, 70, 71, 72–73, 75; lack of, 126; for mealtimes, 58, 60–61, 64; for sleep promotion, 124, 146; for sundowning control, 124; for toileting, 82–83. *See also* scheduling

rummaging, 115

sadness, 34, 51, 105, 106

safety issues: in bathrooms, 82, 90–91; brain trauma avoidance, 144; choking hazards, 38; in the kitchen, 38; in moderate-stage Alzheimer disease, 11

scheduling, 51; exercise, 128; meals, 51, 57, 60; self-care activities, 135; toileting, 82

self-care, 11, 133–39

sensory cues, 27, 48, 52, 58, 89, 126

sensory stimulation / sensory-based knowledge, 2, 25–28, 41–42; in caregivers, 135; with exercise, 107; with favorite activities, 109; multisensory, 37–41; for sundowning control, 124. *See also* auditory stimulation; gustatory stimulation; olfactory stimulation; tactile stimulation; visual stimulation

singing, 89, 90, 107

sleep: brain health effects, 5, 146; environment for, 71–72; required amount, 100

sleep diary, 70

sleep disturbances, 2, 13, 69–77, 91, 141; in caregivers, 149; depression-related, 105; effect of colors on, 32; effect of essential oils on, 35; pain-related, 100; retrogenesis and, 69–71; sleep pattern changes, 69, 70, 75, 99; tips for managing, 71–75, 124

sleep hygiene, 72–73

smell, sense of. *See* olfactory stimulation

smiling, 29, 30

smoking, 141, 142

social interaction, 146

social isolation, 141

solitude, 133

speech deficits. *See* language deficits

speech therapists, 118

spiritual counseling, 108

stimulants, 74

stress management, 128, 134–35

strokes, 142

suicidality, 136

sundowning, 33, 123–25, 129

swallowing difficulties, 13, 56

tactile stimulation, 33, 36; with art, 30–31, 107; attention and concentration effects, 48, 127; for bathing and showering, 89; for bathroom breaks, 82–83; at bedtime, 72, 73; for brain

tactile stimulation (*cont.*)
health, 145; for calming, 125; as communication, 46; cooking as, 37–38; effect on emotions, 25, 26–27, 28; during exercise, 107; during meals, 60, 62–63; for pain management, 100; with pets and other animals, 39; for repetitive behaviors control, 117; for sundowning control, 125; for wandering control, 128
taste buds, 61
tau protein, 4, 5
teeth brushing, 88
temperature, 58, 59, 71, 80
thirst, 91, 117
thought disturbances, 14
time distortion, 12–13, 109, 111
tiredness, 44, 51, 69, 117, 123, 124, 126, 128
toileting, 79–86; before bathing, 91; before bedtime, 73; as repetitive behavior cause, 117; tips for, 80–84
touch. *See* tactile stimulation

under-stimulation, 71, 127
urinary incontinence, 13, 79
urinary tract infections, 82
US Department of Health, *Physical Activity Guidelines for Americans*, 142

verbal communication, 32; of pain, 98, 99; as repetitive behavior, 115, 118; during tasks, 48, 49; tips for, 47–49; tone of voice, 26, 32, 47
verbal cues: for bathing and showering, 88–89, 92; for bedtime routine, 73, 75; for confusion management, 126; during meals, 56, 63–64
vision problems, 56, 81; effect on communication ability, 44, 51; effect on eating ability, 59, 60, 62; in moderate-stage Alzheimer disease, 11, 12; peripheral vision loss, 12, 46, 60, 62, 91
visual cues, 81, 126
visual stimulation, 29–32; with art, 30–31, 107; for bathing and showering, 89, 90; for bathroom breaks, 82–83; cooking as, 37–38; during meals, 60; with pets and other animals, 39
vitamin B deficiencies, 143–44
vitamin C, 144
vitamin D, 144
vitamin E, 144

wandering, 125–29; at night, 69, 70–71, 74–75
weight control, 142
white noise, 72, 118